LAID *AND* CONFUSED

WHY WE TOLERATE BAD SEX
AND HOW TO STOP

MARIA YAGODA

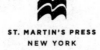

ST. MARTIN'S PRESS
NEW YORK

First published in the United States by St. Martin's Press, an imprint of
St. Martin's Publishing Group

www.stmartins.com

Library of Congress Cataloging-in-Publication Data

Names: Yagoda, Maria, author.
Title: Laid and confused : why we tolerate bad sex and how to stop /
    Maria Yagoda.
Description: First Edition. | New York : St. Martin's Press, 2023. |
    Includes bibliographical references and index.
Identifiers: LCCN 2022058222 | ISBN 9781250277732 (hardcover) |
    ISBN 9781250277749 (ebook)
Subjects: LCSH: Women—Sexual behavior. | Sex (Psychology)
Classification: LCC HQ29 .Y243 2023 | DDC 306.7082—dc23/
    eng/20230111
LC record available at https://lccn.loc.gov/2022058222

Our books may be purchased in bulk for promotional, educational,
or business use. Please contact your local bookseller or the Macmillan
Corporate and Premium Sales Department at 1-800-221-7945, extension
5442, or by email at MacmillanSpecialMarkets@macmillan.com.

First Edition: 2023

10 9 8 7 6 5 4 3 2 1

To the platonic loves of my life

CONTENTS

Our erotic knowledge empowers us, becomes a lens through which we scrutinize all aspects of our existence, forcing us to evaluate those aspects honestly in terms of their relative meaning within our lives. And this is a grave responsibility, projected from within each of us, not to settle for the convenient, the shoddy, the conventionally expected, nor the merely safe.

—*Audre Lorde*

LAID *AND* CONFUSED

INTRODUCTION

I am twenty-eight years old and tired, staring dead-eyed at the condom wrapper in the trash as a man works on my nipples. Reclined on my back, chin propped above his head, I count down from one hundred while his tongue scrambles back and forth between my breasts, the idea of Pleasuring Someone inspiring a sort of mania in him. I lose myself in the vision of the trash can, its contents: a letter from the IRS, a clump of hair from my brush, an empty, family-sized bag of tortilla chips I can't recall eating.

Amid this internal spiral I offer small moans of pleasure, arching my back and grabbing his with a credible enthusiasm that surprises even me. I'm not invested in this man, yet I remain committed to curating a pleasurable experience for him. I resign myself to itemizing trash.

As a longtime sex columnist, I pride myself on my forward-thinking approach to not just sex, but also consent, communication, and pleasure. Yet there I am, tolerating what struck me as cartoonishly bad sex and doing a familiar calculus of "What is easiest?"

Is it easiest to see this through, losing ten-ish minutes of a life I'm not that precious about anyway, and try to glean some validation out of arousing this perfectly pleasant man? Or could I turn this around? Could I say something constructive yet alluring, the way that magazines taught me, something like, "It would be *really* sexy if you stopped growling"? Could I seductively displace his hands, at present squeezing nail-first into my back, and tack them onto my butt, which was crying out for attention?

For years, I've advocated to readers, to friends, and to anyone who will listen in line for the Pret A Manger bathroom that the answer to bad sex is communication. Simply communicate! Don't fake your orgasms. Ask for what you want ☺ ☺ ☺ Now, after years of tedious emotional and scientific research, I'm convinced that it's not so simple.

So, no, I did not speak up. I did not say, "No more nipples," or "It takes me out of the moment when you keep your newsboy cap on." I knew I would never see him again, and communicating with a human person—who is alternately fragile and capable of harm—requires a level of effort that doesn't always feel worth it, when the alternative is simply reclining and waiting, or speeding things up with a fake orgasm, your romantic life already a dazzling web of deceit, so he can ejaculate and you can heat up the pad Thai in your fridge. When the moment to penetrate became obvious—because in a cis-heteronormative society, penetration can feel obvious, inevitable—I performed the requisite choreography.

While now you might be thinking, *How sad and embarrassing for Maria,* as I am, the problem is bigger than my personal poor judgment, as astounding as it may seem. The conceit of this book, and the research supporting it, is that I am not alone in enduring medium bad to very bad sex again and again and again, even though I know better, even though I own good vibrators, even though my therapist is *this close* to leaving the field because I "don't want to be helped."

Regrettably for me, my therapist, and the ever-changing cast of characters I date, my reckoning with bad sex has been gradual and humiliating, like most reckonings that sprawl through your twenties and remain unresolved. The realization that sex is meant to be pleasurable, not a method-acted performance of pleasure so gripping even the actor believes it, sunk in far later than I'd like to admit. But I'll admit it, here, as a public service: my sexual history has been a grand disappointment.

In fact, I am joined by a generation—actually, many generations—of sexually active people who are profoundly dissatisfied with their sex lives and aren't doing much about it, because there are so many other things to take care of, like fighting with health insurance providers and thinking about reading the new Jonathan Franzen.

The Bad Sex Problem is especially noteworthy among millennials and Generation Z, who are famously having less sex than generations before them, a phenomenon known as "the sex recession" that's actually affecting all age groups. Hundreds of young people I've spoken to—of myriad genders, sexualities, and relationship statuses—are experiencing quiet burnout in their sex lives. Experts hypothesize that this "recession"—terminology that suggests there is a healthy, correct amount of sex to have—is fueled by antidepressants, social media, ruinous porn use, and the normalization of getting married later or never at all.

"It's almost like there's a slow-moving, unorganized sex strike of people who can't find good partners or don't desire relationships and are just opting out instead," a twenty-eight-year-old cis straight woman told me.

Personally, I like the sound of that—opting out. The fact that people are having less sex doesn't concern me. So much of sex is horrible! Plus, I strongly disagree that a dip in sexual activity signifies any sort of pathology, when there are perfectly healthy people who desire little sex or, among the asexual community, none at all. What concerns me, rather, is the sex that so many of us *are* having. Many of the factors likely contributing to this "recession," like burnout and endemic loneliness, erode not only our capacity for sexual satisfaction, leading some to opt out, but also our capacity to care about satisfaction itself. In my not-too-distant days of faking orgasms to end sex I found tedious, I suspected I could have better sex if I vocalized "what I wanted," as girl boss culture implores me to. I just didn't care— about my pleasure, about my satisfaction. And there was no guaranteeing my partner would, either.

As much as *Laid and Confused* is a deep dive into the cultural crisis of bad sex, it's also a personal investigation: How and why could a sex expert (me) tolerate such consistently dreadful sex? And how come there are so many others suffering in silence alongside me? What are the social, political, and physical barriers to pleasure that block us from leading affirming sexual lives? The barriers are steep. I feel strongly, however, that working to eliminate, or at least minimize, bad sex from our lives is worth adding to the long list of shit we have to do. Because we are worthy of pleasure, and settling for bad sex can send us a different message.

"What really strikes me about all this research on the sex recession is that it's about the quantity of sex millennials are having, not the quality," Julia Bartz, a New York therapist and author, told me. "If people were having less sex but saying it was more fulfilling, that'd be one thing. But clearly there's a lot of discontent in this area."

There are many obvious socioeconomic factors contributing to sexual discontent. For one: we're tired. Many people in their twenties and thirties report burnout from the constant struggle to yank themselves out of debt without the support of an adequate social safety net. We have multiple side hustles but probably won't own homes. There is also the matter of our poor overstimulated brains. The inability to experience pleasure, a clinical condition known as anhedonia, is on the rise, along with many psychiatric conditions (and treatments) that disrupt sexual satisfaction. And yet, the persistence of bad sex is not strictly about the absence of physical pleasure. We still live in a sex negative society, with abysmal access to inclusive and accurate sex education, and this colors our sexual experiences with shame and confusion. The violent rolling back of reproductive rights, catalyzed by the Supreme Court overturning *Roe v. Wade* (which had guaranteed the constitutional right to an abortion for almost five decades), means that the possibility of forced pregnancy must increasingly factor into the decisions we make around sex. (Of course, abortion access had been abysmal in many parts of the country already and is getting worse with outright bans.) This, too, robs us of pleasure—this full-scale attack on sexual autonomy.

As a birth control–popping, vibrator-hoarding degenerate, I

am indebted to the gains of the sexual revolution of the 1960s, an era credited with normalizing contraception, masturbation, premarital sex, and abortion. Yet decades later, there is something especially striking about the stalled progress surrounding sexual pleasure, even as society grows ever more sex-saturated. In fact, the rollback of abortion rights and a sharp uptick in anti-LGBTQIA+ legislation proves just how nebulous this progress was: our sexual selves remain governed, remain policed.

In *The Right to Sex,* philosopher Amia Srinivasan writes,

> Indeed, what is remarkable about the sexual revolution— this is why it was so formative for the politics of a generation of radical feminists—is how much was left unchanged. Women who say no still really mean yes, and women who say yes are still sluts. Black and brown men are still rapists, and the rape of black and brown women still doesn't count. Girls are still asking for it. Boys still must learn to give it. Whom exactly, then, did the sexual revolution set free? We have never yet been free.

For most of my decade-long sex writing career, and all of my life, I've worked tirelessly to showcase the versions of myself I deemed most attractive. This is standard human stuff— performing—but I suspect I took it further than most. My work to shape a public sexual self that was confident, hot, and self-aware left little space for the authentic sexual self I'm always second-guessing. In my writing, and with romantic partners, I've often felt I had two options, both driven by existential anguish: if I couldn't be pretty, I could be funny, and if I couldn't be funny, I could keep it to myself. I'd resigned myself to a lifetime of bad sex under the condition that I produced goofy anecdotes, or at least hit the dual goals of rehabilitating my self-esteem ("That guy who broke my heart is a loser, ha-ha, he follows NASCAR drivers on Instagram") and entertaining people with events that were not entertaining to me ("He ejaculated onto my eyeballs without asking, ahah?"). Projecting confident fuckability to mask quiet discontent has been a decade-long grift, one that fits neatly into what Rosalind Gill and Shani Orgad call "confidence culture," a contemporary feminism that requires confidence as a prerequisite to empowerment. As a young sex columnist at Yale, I took an assertive stance, writing an article about the ubiquity of bad sex on college campuses that went viral; its opening line, "Guys at Yale are bad in bed." The morning after it was published, I woke to hundreds of Facebook friend requests from men around the country, either asking to fuck me or telling me to die, slut. In the column, I'd positioned myself, and the many women I'd interviewed, as fully formed sexual agents who were being punished by soft dicks at every turn because they didn't ask for "what they wanted"—as if that were something every self-respecting feminist knows from birth. (In reality, women are still punished for expressing sexual desire; rape cases are often dismissed if the victim expresses interest at some point.) A campus celeb who was mentioned in our gossip paper for "sleeping with a sushi waiter for free sushi," a claim only half true, I got a gross little thrill when men recognized me at parties, an increasingly common occurrence; some would approach me to smirk in my vicinity, others to flirt. "You haven't had good sex because you haven't had sex with me," a beefy lacrosse player once told me at a frat house I was quite literally stuck at, my heels tacked to the Natural Light–stained floor.

The radical truth is that in my deeply normal commitment to the bit of being confident and fuckable, I've tiptoed around the ugliness of my sexual history and of bad sex more specifically, doing myself and my readers a disservice. Most of the bad sex we have isn't funny or even that interesting, and we're not always the righteous heroes we believe ourselves to be. Straight men aren't the only reason sex is horrible for so many people, though they certainly put in the work. I've never claimed my sex life was charmed (still, I pray every ex believes it so), but even in my writing about bad sex, I've tended to keep my complicity—and the more mundane, quotidian badness of it—to myself, locked in my skull, where it can rattle around to circus music until I die. I'm embarrassed to know so much about sex, and to have had so much of it, but to still feel so disenfranchised in my sexual relationships, nearly a decade after accusing all men of being sex losers. Yet my reluctance to examine that which I find most embarrassing—total resignation to chronic displeasure—perpetuates the well-documented problem[1] of people believing that everyone else is having better and more sex than them, which makes us mopey about our sex lives, which makes our sex lives worse, which makes us even mopier, and on and on.

This book aims to dispel these myths about other people's sex lives, and to deflate their importance, while we're at it: your sex life is the only sex life that matters. But your sexual problems aren't as personal as they feel. We don't need to feel this great, individual shame, when so many of us are united in it. We've done the best we could with the horrible tools we've been given.

This book proposes better tools. To help make your sex lives more beautiful, more fulfilling, and more not bad, I've put my own sex life on the line, experimenting with practices designed to help us realize our authentic sexual selves, from masturbation meditations to sex cleanses. I hope that one or more of them are useful to you, or at the very least amusing. Sexual healing is not one-size-fits-all, and neither are butt plugs (more on that later). These tools are fundamentally limited, as they call on the individual to adapt, rather than the society that fucked up the individual. But many of the pleasure practices recommended to me by sex therapists, BDSM educators, and even vibrator designers have helped me and others access deeper understandings of our sexualities.

When I talk about bad sex, I am not talking about sex that is shameful, nor am I talking about assault, which is a different kind of bad, and no longer really sex. For the most part, I will avoid discussing assault in my examination of bad, consensual sex, though certainly the fear of assault and the enduring effects of sexual trauma color a lot of these unpleasant encounters. As a survivor of sexual assault, I feel it's important to acknowledge the enduring impact rape and rape culture have on our capacity to enjoy sex. But sex does not have to be assault to be worthy of our scrutiny, and I am interested in unpacking a type of "bad" that I feel is underexamined: the consensual bad.

The badness of bad sex varies wildly. What is enjoyable for one person—role-play that involves accents—is agonizing to me. What is enjoyable for me—role-play that involves charcuterie—is agonizing to someone else. Sexuality is vast and beautiful and goofy! When I say "bad sex" in this book, I am referring to sex that is unsatisfying, non-pleasurable, boring, demoralizing, unfair, depressing, and/or monotonous, whatever that looks like to you. It does not, necessarily, mean that you didn't orgasm. There is an emotional, subjective dimension to good sex that often—but not always—syncs up with orgasm. In fact, too often the outsized emphasis on orgasm sabotages sex entirely, making it outcome-oriented to the point that people are too anxious to enjoy themselves. *"Are you close," he asks me, after a minute of oral.* . . .

So, no, bad sex is not morally wrong; it is simply sex we didn't particularly enjoy, even if our reasons for having it were legitimate. And I am generous with the word "legitimate," because I am serious when I say that bad sex is not shameful, even as we work to avoid it. It is legitimate to sleep with someone because they have good speakers, an amenity you've come to realize you require for watching the *Captain America*s or any Chris Evans film, and sex has sort of just become a part of going to this man's house. I now believe, however, that harmless but disappointing sex has a cost worth considering. Bad sex robs us of time that could have been spent on an activity with a lower physical or emotional toll, like lounging in a towel after a shower. It also sends a signal to ourselves, or maybe confirms a belief we've long held, that our pleasure is not important. If the pleasure of hearing Chris Evans speak so crystal clear that it feels like he's sitting next to you outweighs the pleasure-devoid sex you endured to hear it, so be it. But I want to live in a world where we can feel like Chris Evans is sitting next to us *and* we can enjoy the sex we had before that.

For years, I figured that as long as I used protection and avoided friends' exes, bad consensual sex was a net wash—a silly, aerobic way to pass the time that didn't positively or negatively affect my life. But bad sex is not a wash. It's not a *disaster,* but it's not a wash. In short, bad sex matters because good sex matters. Our pleasure matters. Our eroticism matters. Our time matters. I want to teach myself how to French braid! There is so much I want for me, and for you, that bad sex steals from us; there were so many instances while writing this book that I found myself grieving—for lost energy, lost time, lost spirit, lost self. I ask the question: Why do we tolerate bad sex?, in hopes of moving beyond tolerance, dreaming beyond tolerance, because sexual happiness is a matter of social justice and public health. For those of us who desire sex, sex is good for us. People who report satisfying sex lives feel better in the rest of their lives, and the physical benefits of pleasurable sex, from lower blood pressure to better sleep, are well-documented. Bad sex is worthy of our attention, our scrutiny, because our relationship to pleasure provides innumerable insights into our emotional states, helping us heal and lead fuller, happier lives. For some people, that can mean little sex at all. Pleasure is everywhere.

In her famous 1978 speech, "The Erotic as Power," Audre Lorde talks specifically of the erotic: of the joys that await us when we refuse to settle for the bad, the mundane, in our erotic lives. She imagines what is possible when we prioritize pleasure, rather than settling for lesser sensation, lesser joy. While I wish she were less dismissive of "the pornographic," a category I believe can be enriching, she honors "the erotic" as a valuable source of power that is urgently necessary.

"For once we begin to feel deeply all the aspects of our lives, we begin to demand from ourselves and from our life-pursuits that they feel in accordance with that joy which we know ourselves to be capable of," Lorde wrote. The journey toward "erotic knowledge" that Lorde speaks of is rooted in difficult, at times mortifying, self-interrogation. But when we start asking ourselves what we like and want (orgasms! intimacy! revenge!), we get closer to claiming it. To begin the journey, we must abandon all preciousness. We're talking about mashing and smashing the strangest-shaped parts of our bodies. Sometimes when I'm scraping cum crust off my pillowcase on the way to the hamper, I indulge in daydreams about what might happen if we understood sex as this silly, imperfect thing—not an act to champion or fear. It is not, and cannot be, everything, and this book does not aim to present it as such. I hope to deconstruct sex so we can better understand—and value—our relationship to it: to the bad sex, yes, but also to the sex we love.

SOME NOTES ON METHODOLOGY

This book draws from the most up-to-date research on sexual behavior, from the sociological to the neurological. I have also interviewed hundreds of millennials and Gen Zers about their sex lives, both one-on-one and through anonymous online surveys, and I weave in findings from a decade-long career of interviewing experts and laypeople about sex, while drawing from excruciating personal experiences to contextualize my research. The unfortunate thing about the academic study of sex is just how new and cis-heteronormative it is; the study of queer sexual experiences is limited but growing, which is why official statistics cannot and should not be the only data points.

What's more, sex means different things to different people, which complicates the study of it. So I want to be clear about my working definition of "sex"—its meaning is fluid and deeply subjective, and should never be assumed. Among sexuality professionals there is no consensus on the definition of sex. If that's surprising to you, try to define it yourself, bearing in mind that many people have sex without insertion, orifices, love, or nudity. Is sex any intimate act between two people? Probably not, as that would qualify therapy, asking your stylist for bangs, and passing toilet paper to a stranger. Is kissing sex? Maybe! There's some intimacy and hotness. In her book *The Wheel of Consent,* sex therapist and educator Betty Martin defines sex to mean "the presence of your own arousal and the decision to follow it." I like that. Many sexuality professionals find it more useful to refer to sexual activity or sexual play rather than "sex," which makes space for all the wonderful, kooky shit people enjoy. The broader the definition, the better; limiting the scope of sex limits the pleasure we can feel. In *The Ethical Slut,* an iconic treatise on polyamory from Janet W. Hardy and Dossie Easton, sex is, quite literally, everything:

Sex is anything you do or think or imagine that sets the train in motion: a scene in a movie, a person on the street you think is hot, swelling buds of wildflowers, bursting in a meadow, a fragrance that opens your nose, the warm sun on the back of your head. Then, if you want to pursue these gorgeously sexy feelings, you can increase the swelling tension, and your sensual focus, with any kind of thinking or touching or talking that humans can devise: stroking, kissing, biting, pinching, licking, vibrating, not to mention erotic art and dance and hot music and silky stuff next to our skin.[2]

In this book, I'll be working with a hybrid of Martin's and Hardy/Easton's definitions of sex, but feel free to define it as you please. Like snowflakes and the spots on my Chihuahua's belly, no two sexual experiences look the same, a truth that complicated my project. How could I speak broadly about sex and the people who have it, when there is so much variation among our lived experiences? Is there anything one can even *say* about sex that applies to nearly everyone, regardless of sexuality, gender, race, socioeconomic status, ability, and age? It turns out: yes. Emphatically yes. We all live in bodies that are sexualized, and we are all impacted by cis-heteropatriarchy and purity culture. But my research required moving away from an overreliance on academic studies, which have long marginalized LGBTQIA+ people. In keeping with that, and to prioritize precision, I won't continue the tradition of using the word "woman" as shorthand for cis, heterosexual woman, and "man" as shorthand for cis, heterosexual man. As such, I clarify the sexual and gender identities of people I interview, as they define them and if they felt comfortable sharing that information. I'll share here that I'm nonbinary and have spent most of my sexual life sleeping with men, but my attraction runs the gender gamut. (My gender identity journey is a whole different book that you're welcome to buy later; I won't be excavating that here, because even sex writers can have boundaries.) While including a wide range of gender and sexual identities under an umbrella thesis presented its challenges, I wanted to write a sex book for everyone. Because everyone deserves better sex.

1

THE SEX RECESSION AND
ITS HIDDEN PROMISE

"Sometimes bad sex becomes habitual and I can't break the cycle. Even if physically and mentally it's not enjoyable, on some subconscious level maybe I'm getting something out of it. Vindication? That I'm a 'manly man' and can 'pleasure a woman'? Although if the second part isn't true then, yeah, why continue?"

—*twenty-nine-year-old cis straight man*

I couldn't tell you the exact moment I realized that sex wasn't working for me, but I could tell you the era: post-college, pre-self-realization. I remember taking the subway one night from Bushwick to Manhattan to surprise my then-boyfriend, a tall scientist I didn't particularly care for.

While he was in the bathroom shaving his entire body in that way he did, I crept into his room, where I found a fleshlight lounging on his pillow, its little silicone slit smiling from under a blanket. Panicked, I tried to develop a game plan for his return. Do I acknowledge it? Joke about it? Toss it into that dark wasteland between the bed and the wall? My visceral reaction was disappointment—that my vagina was not enough—and this triggered shame: I was a sex-positive sex writer who at least *intellectually* believed that boyfriends can and should use toys to explore their sexuality. Was I a fraud? Well, yes. But that's a B plot.

He and I hadn't been having sex as often as he might like— just about once a week. I wished it were zero. My clinical depression and the new medication for it worked in tandem to ensure that I was not only incapable of orgasm, but also disgusted by emotional and physical intimacy—cruelly, the only two things I wanted. To pass the time during missionary or doggie style, I'd find an open *New Yorker* on the floor to stare at and rehearse what I'd say to the cable people when I worked up the energy to call them.

"The cable," I'd say, "it never works."

When my boyfriend emerged from the bathroom, his chest gleaming and smooth, I choked. By the time I'd cobbled together a speech about how masturbation was brave and important, he'd thrown the dick tube into his closet and mumbled a defense: we hardly ever had sex. He wasn't wrong, and he didn't owe me an explanation. All genders, no matter their relationship status, should feel empowered to use sex toys. For as many social perks as they enjoy, men are often made to feel ashamed for it.

I told him it was no big deal—that I lovedddd the fleshlight and the fact that he was using one—but the damage was done. The truth was now obvious and awkward: he wished we were having more sex, and I wished we were having no sex. When he broke up with me two weeks later, I felt an unusual lightness, grateful he had made a choice I didn't have the energy to. I slipped into a months-long dry spell that felt cozy and correct, punctuated by masturbation, short-lived dating app flirtations, and sexually charged dreams of Hugh Grant, in character as the villain from *Paddington 2*, taking me out for craft cocktails. The distance from regular, bad sex—which I hadn't even processed as bad because it was so regular—helped me realize that I could, and should, opt out of sex that I hated. Not so coincidentally, I'm part of a generation that's increasingly making the call to have less sex.

There has never been a better time to overhaul our sex lives, and I believe that starts with having less of it, by cutting out the bad stuff and being choosier about the sex we do have. There's good news on that front: studies seem to indicate the millennials—people born between 1981 and 1996[1]—are having less sex than generations before them. Reporter Kate Julian detailed the phenomenon in a viral 2018 *Atlantic* article called "The Sex Recession," which cast a darker light on the trend. There are many theories as to why we're having less sex, the most likely being that several factors are working in tandem: we're burned out, exhausted by a grind that may never drag us out of debt, no matter how many hobbies we monetize; we're on libido-killing antidepressants; we're passing on the nuclear family or marrying later in life; we're eschewing human connection because we're too busy bleep-blooping on our phones. Our attention spans are shot: we can't read two pages of a book, or write two paragraphs of this one, without checking the Instagram of a *Bachelorette* runner-up from seven seasons ago. There's so much porn, truly so much porn, and we can carry it with us wherever we go.

From the late '90s to at least 2016, psychologist Jean M. Twenge found that the average adult went from having sex sixty-two times a year to fifty-four. In her book, *iGen,* she says that people in their early twenties are far more likely to be abstinent than Gen Xers were at that same age. We're seeing this phenomenon around the world, from Japan to Sweden, in various forms, including declining birth rates, and it's affecting all age groups.

Teens are starting their sex lives later,[2] too, and married couples are having less sex than they were a decade ago. Plus, there are more single people than ever before, who are getting married later or never, and singles typically have less sex than people in relationships. As a chronically single individual, I can corroborate this—we simply don't have the access! Coordinating sex takes work, especially when you don't have a live-in partner, which, increasingly, people do not.[3]

The pandemic has accelerated this trend, with all the barriers to sex becoming steeper for pandemic-related reasons; lockdowns, mass death and illness, and widening inequality have not inspired most of us to feel sexual. According to the 2021 General Social Survey, 26 percent of Americans age eighteen and up did not have sex in the past year.

The "sex recession" can still feel deeply paradoxical: not only are young people generally more sex-positive and more educated about safe sex than previous generations, but facilitating sex is the easiest it's ever been. From the comfort of my own toilet, I can coordinate a hookup as mindlessly as I can order my third delivery meal of the day. I can use an app designed for sex and dating, or I can jaunt over to the "other" folder of my Twitter DMs, where a lively assortment of come-ons and penis photos await my consideration. I could set something up with one of those guys! My choices, it would seem, are endless. And yet.

As any depressed person with a vacuum cleaner can tell you, just because an activity seems to require little effort doesn't mean it will happen. Every task I hate—paying bills, going to the pharmacy, scouting sex partners—is streamlined on my phone. Nothing has ever been easier than anything, in the history of everything. And yet, and yet, and yet.

Janet Brito, a sex therapist in Hawaii, told me that while many of her clients who report dissatisfying sex lives are middle-aged, she sees a large contingent of millennials struggling for distinctly millennial reasons.

"They feel connected via social media and don't have the urge to form intimate relationships, as they seem to find fulfillment in other relationships where their emotional needs are getting met," she said. "They are busy pursuing other projects, careers, hobbies, and do not have the time to date—in some cases, due to increased social media communication and having very busy schedules."

At first, her reasoning sounded like yet another way to scold young people for adopting new technology, music, and fashions that rot our brains and erode social mores. But the more I thought about it, the more I realized that, yes, my phone does help sustain the delusion of a vibrant social life. I cobble together small online flirtations—a retweet from a glasses-wearing musician here, a DM from a high school crush there—into a vital imagined romantic life, one that requires far less of me than a real one. I scavenge for that pleasing ding of validation without needing to leave my home to meet a stranger who could be a murderer or five inches shorter than advertised.

For single people, the barriers to sex—namely, putting on pants to meet someone who statistically will disappoint you—steepen with the harassment that often awaits us. There are now thousands of virtual platforms where people can look for love and sex, only to get called ugly sluts or any number of slurs. It makes sense that people would want to opt out. In one study, a third of dating site users said someone sent them sexually explicit photos or messages that they didn't ask for, and a third have also been called explicit names, with 10 percent saying they'd been threatened with physical harm. The toll of being female, LGBTQIA+, and/or BIPOC online is burdensome, on dating apps especially. Lesbian, gay, and bisexual dating app users face more harassment, from name-calling to physical threats, than straight ones.[4] Many queer people report feeling alienated, marginalized, and unprotected by dating apps, despite their very public pushes to promote inclusive branding. Trans Tinder users, for example, still report getting banned arbitrarily.[5]

Apps aside, it's rough out there. Eli Sachse, a forty-one-year-old trans bi man based in Northern California, told me the challenges "start even before having sex and just dating as a trans person. You have to come out as trans at some point, especially if you're going to have sex, but sometimes when you're cruising with gay dudes, they don't even give you that chance." Sachse, a registered nurse, illustrator, and writer, is the author of *Sex Without Roles: Transcending Gender*. "I'll be dancing and a dude will grab for my crotch and not find what he's looking for, and give me a disgusted kind of look like, 'You're fooling me,' that whole kind of thing," he said.

The toll of harassment—and just plain prejudice—feeds into what I believe to be the biggest sex-recessing factor, which is burnout. If you could choose between wading through hundreds of people, some abusive, to find a potential date, *or* lying flat on the floor, recalling that Olympics where Bob Costas's pink eye got progressively worse, which would you choose? To rest, or to suffer?

The slew of tiny exertions required to orchestrate sex—say, perusing Grindr half asleep or kissing your long-term boyfriend's neck—feel more daunting with each passing day. Everything feels daunting now, for millennials, it seems. We're the "burnout generation," and efficiency isn't the cure.

Quite tragically, sex requires a wealth of physical and emotional energy. Sex feels like yet another item on the long list of things we should be doing, which renders it ever more daunting, in a way that passively sinking into forty episodes of *The Nanny* never will. The millennial burnout theory paints a bleak picture of the "sex recession"—it suggests that our reticence to have sex stems from a profound lethargy you can only embody when you know you'll never be able to afford retirement. *I find this explanation compelling,* I type from my bed before closing my laptop for my 3 P.M. Depression Nap.

"I think having more sex would be nice. If time permitted, I'd definitely try to make it happen on Grindr or Tinder," a thirty-year-old cis gay man told me. "But as I'm getting older, I feel like I've been hedging a lot more. Like, is it worth risking having sex with someone who ends up being terrible? Maybe I should just jack off on my own and call it a night."

Hey, that sounds like a nice night. The dip in sexual activity is not all bleak, even if some of the factors causing it are. Many theorize that declining birth rates in many countries reflect a broader uptick in freedom available to childbearing people. So fewer people are getting married? Fantastic. Studies have shown that married straight women, for one, often report feeling coercion from their husbands to have sex. Women are raising their relationship standards so significantly "that dating opportunities for heterosexual men are diminishing," claimed a recent *Psychology Today* article that urges men to address their skills deficits. Let's fucking goooo.

New research[6] even indicates that people who have no desire to marry report better sex lives than single people who want to eventually marry, proving, at least a little, the toxicity of the heteronormative nuclear family—even the idea of it—as it relates to sex.

The broadening of choices chronicled by social scientists benefits everyone, but particularly women and the LGBTQIA+ community. Crucially, increased freedom to opt out of marriage and monogamous, cis-heteronormative sexual arrangements improves the quality of life for asexual people, who represent around 1 percent of the American population (many experts agree that this estimate is conservative). Asexual people do not experience sexual attraction, but can be romantically attracted to all genders—sub-categories include biromantic, heteromantic, and aromantic.

Julie Kliegman, a nonbinary writer who came out as asexual,

or ace, in 2016, spent a giant chunk of her life having sex she didn't like. It wasn't until she saw an episode of *BoJack Horseman,* where a primary character reveals he is asexual, that she reconsidered her sexual history and put the pieces together: sex was not for her, at all.

"I knew I didn't care for it exactly, but I didn't know that it was an option to opt out of it altogether," she said. To the extent she dates at all ("It's rough out there"), Kliegman seeks intimate, romantic relationships with people of all genders that don't include sex. As asexual representation increases, she suspects more people will come out and stop having sex. This is a fantastic thing, even though it would technically fall under the umbrella of the sex recession.

"A lot of people are puzzling through how they feel about sex," she said, "and I think the asexuality label might apply to some of them."

I refuse to accept the sex recession as another depressing facet of our generation. In fact, I celebrate it—we've been given an unprecedented opportunity to reevaluate our relationship with sex, which, for some, looks like abandoning it entirely. The *actual* depressing thing is not how little sex we're having; it's how much bad sex we're having.

☙ ❧

Plenty of young people have found relief in sex-recessing. One twenty-seven-year-old cis straight woman I spoke with told me that her recent hiatus from sex and dating—a realm that has been consistently disappointing for her—has dramatically improved her mental health.

"I deleted all my apps, and wanted a break from dating in general. I didn't want to go out of my way to go on dates for the sake of dates, but wanted it to feel more intentional and focus on myself, my friends, my work," she said. "Now I'm still doing all those same things, and while I miss physical contact, it does feel liberating to not be defined by my dating life, but my own interests. My head feels clear, and it's nice to focus my energy on other things. It was interesting and a little frightening to see how much brain space dating took up."

Unplanned ebbs in sex and dating, however, can be distressing to some, especially those who've internalized norms about how much sex is "healthy" or "enough." The conversation surrounding the sex recession, which suggests that there is a normal amount of sex people should have (there's not), feeds these anxieties. One of the many barriers people face to sexual satisfaction is the heavy, shameful feeling that their sex lives aren't as orgasmic or spontaneous or jam-packed as their peers'.

"We are filled with expectations that are unrealistic," sex therapist Jessa Zimmerman told me. "We think we must be broken; there must be something wrong with us. It's very isolating."

A major part of therapy for Lindsay, a thirty-one-year-old cis queer woman, has been rethinking her relationship with sex and her body, and a major part of *that* has been rethinking sexual frequency. A lifelong source of relationship anxiety for her has been: *Am I having enough sex? And if not, is it because I am undesirable?* When we spoke, Lindsay had been dating a woman for a year and a half, and the drop-off in sex once the pandemic started triggered her anxieties about hitting the correct number of fucks per week to feel confident in the relationship. In recovery for an eating disorder, she is working to unlearn this intense scrutiny of her physical state, including her sex life.

"I still really put sex on a pedestal so that I can feel okay with my physical body," she said. "I definitely felt bummed when the frequency dropped." She recalled a conversation from early in her relationship when her partner said that in past dating experiences, she'd have sex two or three times a week. "I thought, 'Oh my God, am I a terrible partner?'"

Lindsay has been trying to practice radical acceptance. "I'm not necessarily fixated on the frequency now, but just how it feels—you know, the quality versus quantity," she said. "I feel like when you're trying to just check the box for sex this week, it feels so transactional and gross. It feels like we're doing it so that we can like tell everyone, 'We're okay! We're still having sex!' So, it's just been about trying to take that pressure away."

Most people I've interviewed who are unsatisfied with their sex lives cited anxiety about the disconnect between the amount of sex they had and the amount they felt they were supposed to have. They felt their number wasn't high enough, but didn't necessarily want to have more, either. While low sexual activity can sometimes be a cause for concern—say, in the case of an otherwise horny person whose new meds eviscerate her sex drive—the preoccupation with prescribed numbers is a recipe for a) shame when you don't hit them, and b) bad sex when you force yourself to.

I welcome the sex recession as a reset—a moment to reconnect with our authentic sexual desires, rather than the ones prescribed to us, that can look like stepping away from sex altogether (at least until we figure out what's going on).

"We've entered a minefield of new pressures to appear and act free and empowered, and these pressures to perform are out of sync with—and exacerbate—our own internal disquiet," writes anthropologist Katherine Rowland in *The Pleasure Gap*. "The outward display of boldness, sexiness, the eager libertine, may have little relation to the anxiety, self-censorship, and pleasure neglect contained within."

If the claims of a "sex recession" are true, if young people are having less sex than any generation before them, then we're ideally positioned to harness the power of opting out of sex we don't want to have and make space for the sex we do.

≈ ≈

I remember the first time I opted out of sex that would have been bad. I succeeded in this instance and then somehow *Eternal Sunshine*'d the memory, as I would go on to have bad sex repeatedly for years to come. Figuring out the appropriate way to say no is an ongoing process, and the horrible news is we must do it all on our own, failing repeatedly. The medium news is you get better each time you practice reclaiming your sexual agency.

I was twenty-one and had just moved to Brooklyn. I was wasted, floating back from a night at some West Village bar/club, waiting for the train that would take me to the L that would take me to my tiny room in East Williamsburg by the Brooklyn-Queens Expressway. There I would often fantasize about jumping from my lofted bed onto the wooden floor, hoping to injure myself just enough to get out of work but not enough to be hospitalized. I was a sandwich maker at a café for affluent people by the river. I sliced deli meats and spread harissa aioli and pickled beets until my calves ached, flecks of ham gathering in my bra, all to sustain an unpaid magazine internship and some weekend nights out where I hoped to have sex with someone rich enough to buy me drinks but not rich enough to fetishize my lifestyle.

The bar/club, notorious for the horniness of its clientele, had not been fruitful that night. I had acquired the number of a jovial man who, to this day, is listed in my phone as "Greek the Club," but I'd reached the point of the night where something shifted in me physically and moved me toward home.

But swaying on the subway platform, a little past midnight, I caught eyes with a man across the tracks who seemed tall. I was still feeling flirty in my Forever 21 bandage skirt and disintegrating black combat boots, and he was clearly still feeling flirty in his, well, couldn't see that far, there were two tracks between us and my contact lenses had expired years ago. But we waved at each other and alternated looking down coyly.

Feeling bold, I mimed out my number with my hands—Four. Eight. Four—and he typed it into his phone. Just as I finished the last digit my train whooshed down the tracks, and I floated to the next station. When my service returned, I received his text and texted back my address, telling him to come over. He was a firefighter visiting a friend from out of town, I learned. As I trudged down Graham and my buzz continued its march toward exhaustion, I tucked my phone into my purse, acquired a bodega bacon egg and cheese, and slipped into bed with it. Twenty minutes later, brushing miscellany like assorted pencils and sandwich foil off my sheets, I spotted my phone lighting up out of the corner of my eye. "I'm here." Who the hell? What? Oooooooohhhhhh.

I peered out my street-level window and an entire human man was standing there. I didn't recognize him. Then the night came trickling back like a cinematic montage of girls on Molly: lights, Greek the Club, Jägerbombs, Flo Rida, hobbling across Meatpacking cobblestones, subway, Four. Eight. Four.

I texted him that I was so sorry but very tired. He said please can I come in. I said I am tired but so sorry. He said, I came all this way. At this point I was wearing a bra and no bottoms. I slipped into sweats and ran out, grateful that I had done a bad job taking off my makeup because it still mattered to me to look pretty. He seemed nice, but I did not want to have sex with him. I'd reached a point in my life where I was *considering* not having sex with people when I didn't feel like it.

Feelingly horrible that he had traveled all this way—to be clear, fifteen minutes by taxi—I let him make out with me by my door. This was my way of apologizing for not having sex with him, my own mouth offered as consolation. He kept lobbying to come inside. I kept saying I was tired, and he kept saying he could come in just for a little, that he wouldn't take very long. I kept offering more make-out to apologize. The cycle continued. After fifteen minutes or an hour, I worked up the resolve to pull away, bid a firm adieu, and stepped back inside, locking the door. If I had been one-eighth less tired, if one of the drinks Greek the Club bought me had been a vodka Red Bull and not a tequila soda, I would have had drunken intercourse with that stranger because he "had come all that way" and seemed disappointed, and from a young age I learned it is my job to manage people's feelings. Not only did I have to fend off pressure from the firefighter, but my internal sense of "compulsory sexuality"—the social pressure to have sex and be sexual in situations you don't want to have sex or be sexual—implored me to invite him in. It easily could have gone the other way.

In the near decade since hurting that man's feelings, I haven't entirely shaken the impulse to emotionally caretake via sex, a sentiment that has been echoed to me by many people in relationships who feel burned out in their sex lives. It can feel like sex is something to be offered or withheld, rather than wholeheartedly enjoyed.

But I want to give myself, and all of us, credit for the bad sex we have managed to avoid—those instances we listened to our gut and mustered up the energy to resist what felt like an inevitable sequence of events. If the sex recession has us scaling back on sex we don't feel like having, we should celebrate it.

2

THE BAD SEX PROBLEM

"An anthropologist visiting our planet might conclude that ours is a culture gluttonous for pleasure and sexually ravenous. And yet, what I observe daily in my clinical practice is that for all of this pleasure-seeking behavior, all of this wanting of pleasure, very few of us seem able to fully experience the sensations or satisfaction we seek."

—Nan Wise, PhD, Why Good Sex Matters

When I was twenty-two, I was certain there was nothing left for me in Brooklyn. I quit my job, sold all my things, and fled to Naples, Italy, a dreamy, smelly place where postlunch naps feel legally mandated. After a monthslong stretch of fighting for a visa and building a robust social circle of seniors and pizza men, I had to flee again, because of the law. I packed a large, military-grade backpack, gifted to me by a lovestruck middle-aged man named Biagio, and took an overnight ferry to Split, Croatia. (The tattered bag was from the war, he said; I never learned which one.) Once I settled in a small village outside of the city, and my body acclimated to a diet of cabbage, smooth sausages, and supermarket wine, I met a man with a long fluffy ponytail at an underground club, or a club that felt underground to me, darkened with smoke and off-brand grunge. After flirting in simple English about whether my life in New York had been like *Friends* ("Is Joey real??" he asked), I went home with him, we started hooking up, and, somewhat abruptly and without negotiation, he ejaculated on my face. It stung. He handed me tissues to dab the fluids and then slipped into a soft pajama onesie, ready for bed. I didn't think much of the experience, only that I had an interesting story to relay to friends and, one day, readers.

A few weeks later, after shaving off half my hair to establish I was misunderstood, I met a tall, handsome cruise ship worker at the same club and brought him home to my rental apartment. We sat on the stony stretch of Adriatic that was my backyard; the sea was inky black. He kept asking me if I'd seen *Californication,* and reciting lines from it that I found inscrutable, as he was translating the Croatian translation back into English. Hooking up with him felt exciting and odd. The make-out was frenetic as we tore off each other's clothes, knocking over abandoned water glasses left and right. I asked him to get a condom. He refused; he said he could not have sex with a condom, that it was agonizing for him. So we didn't have sex. We simply laid there on the bed, each of us hoping the other would fold; people had clearly folded to him before. (His jawline could have sliced an apple.) But unprotected sex with a stranger was off-limits to me. He continued trying to convince me to forgo the condom, citing low pregnancy rates. This is when I should have sent him home. After explaining the premise of *Californication* again, he hoisted himself up from the bed and peed into the sink, looking at me through the mirror as he did it. A few nights later, head throbbing from supermarket wine, I invited him back.

For years, retelling these stories to myself and others, I'd recall the first sexual encounter as bad and the second one as good, sexy, and fun—a disturbing testament to the skill with which I cling to scraps of intrigue to fill the void. The first guy was textbook inappropriate, and I was textbook unattracted to him, from the tip of his ponytail to the butt flap of his onesie. He used me as a prop for his satisfaction, and I complied, sustained by novelty and an eagerness to feel something, anything. The second guy was stoic and aggressive in a way that aroused me, despite his rudeness around condoms, which I too quickly brushed aside. In both cases I understood there was a possibility I could be killed and didn't care; in both cases, I understood I wouldn't get off and didn't care. In that era of my life, sex hadn't been about pleasure. It was a means to feel desired and less alone. And it didn't even work!

My bar was low. My bar was "ideally not murdered but not so bad if murdered." Eventually, I returned to New York City to rebuild the life I'd blown up when I moved to Naples. I continued to label my Croatian sexploits, just as I always had, as either horrible or fantastic—an impulse that in many ways reflects the black-and-white thinking around sex that haunts our society. The men marked two ends of the casual sex spectrum that fit neatly into storytelling, which for a time was the most useful part of my sexual encounters. Writing about sex helped convince me my dalliances were worth something, even if they meant nothing to me. I'd long passed the point where such kooky adventures could be considered character-building, so at least I could get a paycheck and publicly scold the men who'd ejaculated on my eyeballs.

For many people, this is part of growing up—not dabbing cum off their lashes, but having bad sex until they figure out what good sex is. It takes some longer than others to distinguish between the two. Without any real success in the long-term relationship department, I missed some of the opportunities that allow you to figure out what good sex means to you personally, which often happens in a relationship with someone you trust. I thought sex with the cruise ship worker was good because I thought he was hot, and that it was hot that he thought I was hot, and it felt important to me that, having fled two countries in the night that year, I have hot sex with Croatian strangers who could affirm the deranged coming-of-age bender I was on. But sex is never just sex, just like fleeing is never just fleeing. We use sex— bad sex—to solve personal problems, and it usually doesn't work.

However personal it may feel—and, fuck, it feels personal— bad sex is one of the oldest customs in human history. Much like stone tools and shells as currency, bad sex is mundane, utilitarian. Our tools have grown more sophisticated, and shells have found their way onto the necklaces your dad buys on vacation, but bad sex endures, quietly.

While I can't personally speak to the quality of sex several millennia ago, it is safe to assume it was bleak, given what we know now about what people knew then about sex. I'll start with the Greeks: Aristotle believed that sperm was excrement. Archilochus, a lyric poet from the seventh century BC who was famous for his erotic verses, also paints a somewhat unfortunate picture. In one of his steamier bars, he likens sex to a quotidian farm transaction: "His penis is swollen / like a donkey from Priene / taking his fill of barley."[1] (In another poem, his depiction of arousal has been translated both as "boil in the crotch" and "feeble now are the muscles in my mushroom.")

We can go back further, even, to ancient Mesopotamia. A remarkable Babylonian clay plaque[2] depicts a man fucking a woman from behind as she drinks beer through a straw—she's unbothered by the sex, but more focused on the beverage. (There are, surprisingly, many artistic riffs[3] on the trope of Man Penetrating Woman While She Drinks Through a Straw, dating to around the first and second millennia BC. Petition to bring back drinking beverages during boring sex.)

Of course, sex has always been pleasurable *enough,* useful *enough,* for people to continue having it and populating the species. To be fair, there are loads of centuries-old pieces of art and literature that are hot (see, Sappho, Giulio Romano, and shunga art from Japan's Edo period). But my suggestion that sex has been tolerated, rather than enjoyed, by many people throughout human history is not a leap.

"What is it that we demand of sex, beyond its possible pleasures, that makes us so persistent?" mused philosopher Michel Foucault in *The History of Sexuality,* volume 1, a work that I return to repeatedly in my quest to understand how we, humanity, got so absolutely deranged about sex, so obsessed with sex that we would have bad sex again and again and again.

👁 👁

All the social developments that have made sex easier—dating apps, birth control, a carte blanche from the sex-positivity movement (or was it the body pos movement?) to never shave my genitals—haven't moved the dial on better. Bad sex has endured. Young people may be better at discerning good sex from bad sex, in part thanks to resource-sharing on platforms like TikTok and Instagram, but not necessarily getting closer to having it. I'm a professional sex writer who is labia-deep in the latest research on maximizing pleasure, communicating with partners, and feeling sexually confident, yet most of the sex I've had has landed somewhere between passable and "huh."

And it's not just me, or because I'm single, having one-off encounters where both parties are too intoxicated or unobligated to reasonably deliver. The persistence of boring, unsatisfying, uncomfortable sex is top of mind for many sex therapists, social psychologists, journalists, and academics.

"Sex is no better now than it was when I was in high school," sex therapist Jessa Zimmerman told me. "There might be more about consent now, but it's still not talked about, and we are not equipped to talk about it . . . I don't think we're any more equipped now than we were in the fifties."

The '50s?? When sitcom couples slept in different beds? Man. So much has improved since then—sitcoms, haircuts, the taste of liquid medicine—so why not sexual pleasure? For one, I can watch any kind of porn anywhere at any time, even inside of this self-serious Brooklyn coffee "lab" where I'm writing this. For two, men are constantly explaining to me that they "actually like going down on women." What's gone so, so wrong?

Neuroscientist Dr. Nan Wise, author of *Why Good Sex Matters,* suggests we are up against unprecedented obstacles, the biggest one being "the pleasure crisis." Citing skyrocketing rates of anhedonia, Wise posits that the ever-increasing external stimuli in our environments, and the "bombardment of easy-to-access, seemingly endless supply of quick-fix pleasures," are not conducive to feeling more of anything, let alone satisfaction.

In many ways, we've gone backward from the sexual revolution of the 1960s; rather, we're still enduring the backlash to it, argues historian Dagmar Herzog in her ever-relevant 2008 book *Sex in Crisis,* which traces America's sex anxiety to the legislative victories of conservative evangelicals.

"Our national conversation about sex now suffers a tremendous impoverishment," Herzog writes. "It is fairly easy to find information about how to have sex or techniques for how to improve sex. It is simple to find near-frenzied talk about adolescents' exposure to sexual imagery on the internet or alarm over teens' potentially risky behavior. It is far tougher to find frank and open dialogue about our hopes and fears for our children's—and our own—sexual health and happiness. There is much titillating talk about sex in America, yet there is very little talk about sex that is morally engaged and affirmative." (More than fifteen years later, Herzog's analysis rings truer every day, with a dizzying uptick in legislative efforts to police adolescent sexuality and gender identity, particularly in schools.)

Over a decade after her book, the lack of sex-positive, pleasure-minded public discourse on sexual wellness is fucking dark, to put it mildly. When it comes to sexual happiness, we're still left to fill in the blanks, seeking out our own information from popular culture that so often leads us astray (for instance, presenting synchronized orgasm as the norm).

Desperate for *some* evidence of progress while researching this book, I caught up with Maria Trumpler, a Yale professor of gender and sexuality studies who was my advisor when I was a horny, miserable undergraduate sex columnist. During the pandemic, Trumpler was stationed at her home in Vermont, where she makes cheese and teaches undergraduate courses remotely. One such course is "Food, Identity, and Desire," which explores the intersections of appetites and identity. Trumpler's students are what we would call "Gen Z"—people born in the late '90s and early 2000s. It's been over ten years since I was in college, routinely sleeping with a classmate I didn't get along with and bingeing children's cereal on nights I wasn't drunk enough to text him. I asked Professor Trumpler if her students were still having horrible sex, even though we are ten years in the future, even though they are better connected and educated than I ever was, even though they know more about the politics of gender identity, sexuality, and consent.

Trumpler, who has taught a first-year seminar on the history of sexuality for nearly twenty years, pointed out that her students don't often talk to her about their sex lives. But she said that pleasure, in general, remained fraught for them, if not outright taboo, and this extends beyond sex.

"My first-years so often don't take pleasure in their bodies or in sex, and don't take pleasure in food," she said, noting that the people who take her courses are exceptionally sex-positive. "Often they're people who really have learned that the way to succeed is by tamping down their experiences of pleasure and focusing on long-term goals." Of course, Trumpler is observing a very specific segment of the population—Yale undergraduates do not, and I can't emphasize this enough, represent America—but the disconnect between her students' experience of sex-positivity and sex happiness is revealing. In fact, in part due to this growing malaise, plenty of Gen Zers are abandoning the ideals of sex-positivity all together; in one recent *BuzzFeed* article, Gen Z women called it "passé" and "corny."[4]

So, yes, people may be more fluent in the language of sexuality than generations before them—which matters—but they are having so much unsatisfying sex, and are so profoundly resigned to it, if they haven't abandoned sex entirely. Amplified by the internet (thanks a million!), the harmful social pressures that form the backdrop of our sexual identities all but guarantee a cultural climate of bad sex.

Over the course of hundreds of interviews with sexually active millennials and Gen Zers, I've found that sexual dissatisfaction is nondiscriminating, plaguing both people in relationships and single folks like me, who sleep with an ever-rotating lineup committed enough to DM garlic bread memes but not enough to spare a toothbrush. Regardless of relationship status, we face unique sexual roadblocks.

For people in relationships, bad sex often looked like middling, boring intimacy upkeep. Among both camps, bad sex serves a specific purpose, even when it is not pleasurable. A twenty-eight-year-old cis woman who identifies as "hetero-ish" said that sometimes sex with her partner is just "maintenance." Maintenance sex is wildly common among people in romantic partnerships.

"It's the days where maybe neither my boyfriend nor I feel super excited about having sex, but it's sort of an acknowledgement of our mutual attraction and maintaining intimacy, playfulness, or whatever," she said. "There are times when it's not balanced—

like he will be more eager to have sex or vice versa, and I want to be game even if I am not as excited by the prospect."

A thirty-one-year-old cis gay man told me something similar. "If it's something I did for him, then I'm ultimately glad it happened because that kind of intimacy is important for all of us," he said. "I can tell that the times we get short and easily rattled with each other are usually because we haven't been intimate in a while, and when we do I definitely notice a positive difference in mood."

Then there is bad sex among single people, wherein lack of comfort and familiarity is one of the biggest issues. In fact, bad sex with one-off partners is among the most laughably bad, I am devastated to report, and my upstairs neighbor can regrettably corroborate.

"I'd say most of the casual, consensual sex I've had was in the meh to bad range," a twenty-eight-year-old cis straight woman told me. "A few common features include jabby fingering, lackluster oral where it feels like they want to do it for points but don't actually have a technique, and flipping me over every two seconds because they watch a lot of mainstream porn where shots are fifteen seconds long so staying in one position feels too boring."

The party line among sex therapists is that good sex comes with practice and a level of comfort that's difficult to cultivate with strangers, though many people do—plenty of people in the non-monogamy community told me that casual sex is the most pleasurable for them. If you're in a relationship, and you *do* have the perceived advantage of emotional connection, you can easily fall into sexual ruts that feel way too exhausting to climb out of. We're tired! Did you know that human green-house gas emissions are responsible for thousands of deaths each year? There are so many things to worry about. I'm not suggesting we worry about sex—anti-choice political leaders, select youth pastors, and our parents do enough of that for us—but rather, that we consider investing some of our (lim-ited) energy into understanding the root causes of our sexual dissatisfaction so we can feel less of it.

CULPRIT 1: ANHEDONIA

Numerous studies suggest that young people are experiencing growing rates of anhedonia, or the reduced motivation and capacity to feel pleasure, and the pandemic made things con-siderably worse across all populations.[5] The term encapsulates a wide range of deficits in hedonic function, including major disruptions to the neural pathways that enable us to want and like things. Some researchers cite this anhedonic wave as one of the core phenomena fueling the sex recession, as it becomes harder to justify the work of coordinating sex when the experi-ence doesn't even feel pleasurable.

Anhedonia is a principal symptom of many mental health conditions that are spiking in recent years, including substance abuse, major depression, and personality disorders.[6] Recent studies show an alarming rise in psychological pain across all age groups, genders, races, and socioeconomic statuses, includ-ing a steep rise in clinical anxiety and depression, which share anhedonia as a common clinical feature.[7] In one study, the

American Psychological Association found the rise in mental health disorders over the past decade to be particularly severe among young adults, with increased use of digital media hypothesized as a driving factor.[8]

Then the pandemic happened. The broad increase in mental health issues and psychological pain has only steepened during COVID-19; in 2020, the CDC shared that the percentage of Americans reporting symptoms of anxiety disorder has increased roughly threefold compared with the same period in 2019, with a rise in anxiety, depression, and suicidal ideation highest among adults aged eighteen to twenty-four.[9]

In a cruel turn of events, many of the medications prescribed to treat these conditions make arousal and orgasm extremely difficult. In tackling the central nervous system, SSRIs can affect other neurotransmitters and hormones involved in sex, including testosterone and dopamine. I cannot tell you how many times I've had intercourse with a man for what feels like thirty hours, only for him to tell me at hour thirty and one minute that he's on Lexapro so he can't come but is having a blast. Usually, I'm the one flaunting the sexual side effects of medication. I've been on Prozac and other meds for major depression for almost half of my life. These drugs have made orgasming with a partner even more difficult for me, a chronically fatigued depressive who is insecure about approximately five major body parts. While I know orgasm cannot and should not be the arbiter of good sex—and that the pressure to orgasm adds undue anxiety—I have found it difficult to unlearn the outsized importance that's been placed on it by society. Also, orgasming feels good! It is okay to want to orgasm during sex.

On a neurobiological level, anhedonia blocks our natural biochemical responses to activities that are wired to give us joy, like exercise, social relationships, and sex. It prevents us from fully letting go into excitement, playfulness, and curiosity—basically everything that makes sex enjoyable and satisfying.

Anhedonia is not the sole culprit for the Bad Sex Problem, but it steepens the biochemical barrier to entry (ayyy). If we're already more likely to have difficulty feeling pleasure, we stand less of a chance against the other forces conspiring to ensure sex is a drag or worse, a slog. Not to be all "society!!" but social forces have further complicated our relationships to the pleasure we are already struggling to feel. So, yes, society!!

CULPRIT 2: SEX EDUCATION

We have more information at our disposal than in any other era of human history.

While in line at the supermarket, I can search "is my labia wrong" and peruse 4.1 million results. One problem with this bounty of information, though, is the deluge of unvetted garbage.

As I search for labia solutions, the algorithm serves me many science-based resources that assure me crooked-looking labia are no cause for concern, but also an Australian government website[10] that suggests taking baths is bad for your labia, and *that* is what will lodge betwixt my brain folds forever. Even when I'm not actively looking to validate labia insecurities, labia insecurities find me in my own home! Ads for labiaplasty regularly splash on my browser as I labor to read the news or shop for sweaters. (It's no wonder that the number of people seeking surgery to alter the appearance of their labia has skyrocketed in the past five years. The same is true of ball-enhancing procedures.)

Sensitive and easily agitated, I am vulnerable to this kind of messaging about my genitalia, but I'm not as vulnerable as adolescents, who are more likely to internalize these cues long-term, in part because their brains are squishier. What we learn about sex, bodies, and pleasure during our development has a lasting impact on the way we experience sex. Therein lies the problem: sex education in America remains inaccurate or non-existent, and the other institutions that teach us about sex— like family, church, and mass media—are largely reinforcing cis-heteronormative, puritanical values that marginalize our most vulnerable youth and interfere with their sexual well-being. Too often these institutions stigmatize sexual pleasure, perpetuating messages like: sex is scary; genitals are gross; sex is for men's pleasure; sex is straight; sex is intercourse; sex is ejaculation; sex is for certain types of bodies (read white, cis, straight, and thin). Around the country, school boards and lawmakers are instituting bans on books dealing with race, gender, and sexuality at an unprecedented pace, and books written by Black and LGBTQIA+ authors are under disproportionate attack.[11]

As psychotherapist and relationship genius Esther Perel puts it in *Mating in Captivity,* "[I]t is in messages to children that societies most reveal their values, goals, incentives, prohibitions." How can you have good, passionate, pleasurable sex when these messages still live inside you, messages that say the sex you are having is wrong, and that you are wrong for having it?

A growing body of research shows that sex education is more effective at promoting health when it's pleasure-inclusive.[12] When mortified parents or health teachers teach us about sex, however, they usually fail to point out that sex is supposed to feel *good*. At school, talking points stick to the risks of sexual activity, like STIs and unwanted pregnancy. If we're jackpot lucky, and find ourselves in a classroom that acknowledges birth control, we're given the opportunity to roll a condom atop a banana dick. But even in more progressive classrooms, pleasure rarely comes up. The genitalia on worksheets tend not to have significance beyond reproduction or dick insertion. The gender-essentialist framing of sex ed, which often begins with a division of the boys and the girls to teach half-baked lessons on wet dreams and menstruation, leaves us entirely on our own to figure out pleasurable, affirming sex in a culture stacked to deprive us of it. So, porn becomes our sex ed. Our idiot friends become our sex ed. Racy teen soaps become our sex ed.

Maybe it makes sense that the middle school gym teachers of America don't want to teach adolescents about the benefits of jacking off, or that most clitoris-having people can only orgasm from clitoral stimulation, rather than penetrative sex. And it makes sense that parents of adolescents might feel odd about their kids getting this information at school. Insidious social discomfort with sexuality is nothing new, going back *at least* two millennia, though popping off with the Puritans and, then, the Victorians.

Harmful and/or wrong information about sex may not be new, but it has grown exponentially more impactful: the media we stare at throughout the day, whether TikTok or Pornhub or hour seventy of a *Sister Wives* binge, has amplified our exposure to toxic messaging. Laurie Mintz, a professor of human sexuality at the University of Florida and author of *Becoming Cliterate,* suspects that millennials and Generation Zers are the most sexually misinformed generations of all time, given the unprecedented accessibility of misinformation.

"They have more false images than we ever did," Mintz told me. "I'm not against porn, but the problem with it is when it is widely available and sexual education is not, and lessons in porn literacy are not."

One example, Mintz said, is "socializing women that if it's good for him, it's good for [her]." Sex ed has not sufficiently leveled up to counter these messages. We're outnumbered.

"At best, the girls are told about their period. At worst: 'Stay a virgin, or you're going to die,'" said Mintz. "The only message and models they have for sex are women who have fast and fabulous orgasms with, you know, two minutes of warm-up. When they try that, it's not only unpleasant, but it hurts. And instead of thinking, 'Ooh, I better go get some information,' they say, 'Something's wrong with me,' and suffer in silence. They're so indoctrinated with the false images."

The easy abundance of "false images" makes sex ed even more important, and yet it fails us so profoundly. Maya Williams, a queer nonbinary poet and activist, remembers the sex ed in their hometown being "super clinical" and overwhelmingly white. "What was fascinating to me was whenever anatomical graphs were used, regardless of the majority population at the school, it was always a white body being displayed," they told me. "It was like, 'Oh, I don't see myself in this equation. I don't see Black people engaging in sex.'"

I began researching this book with the assumption that sex education had improved over the past several decades. I now realize this was delusional. I tend to assume that, for the most part, the more time that passes, the better things get. While this has been true of my back acne, it has not been true of American sex education.

In public school classrooms, children are still exposed to scientifically inaccurate, homophobic, transphobic, racist, and fear-based sex education, if they're exposed to anything at all. According to the Guttmacher Institute, only seventeen states require sex education content to be medically accurate. What's more, nineteen states *require* in-school instruction on the importance of saving yourself for marriage, and twenty-nine states *require* that abstinence be the focus of the curriculum.[13]

I now feel enormously grateful that the only thing I can recall from sex ed was getting tossed free deodorant and thick, off-brand pads. Curious about the scope of the American sex ed crisis, I asked my Twitter followers to share the most wrong, most offensive things they were taught about sex in school. The responses were chilling. I'm listing a few here so I don't have to be alone with them, and to underscore how perfectly reasonable it is that people still have fraught relationships with sexual pleasure.

"If you swallow cum a weird cauliflower-looking fungus would grow in your throat and suffocate you to death within days."

"Women don't actually enjoy sex; they only enjoy the closeness and intimacy."

"At a certain point during sex, men 'can't stop and have to keep going' even if the woman says to stop."

"You might be able to get HIV via enthusiastic French kissing."

"I was told that sex was like chewing gum. And you know what happens to gum? It gets spit on the ground, because no one wants someone else's chewed-up piece of gum. Which was super cool to hear as a survivor of sexual trauma."

"Sex is binary, and everyone is always labeled correctly at birth."

"I was told that women are like stickers and if you put down a sticker and pull it off, it won't be as nice when you try to put it down again."

"STIs are death sentences and gay sex is a footnote."

"I had an abusive conservative parent that wouldn't sign the permission slip allowing me to receive sex education in the first place."

"Nothing. Nothing about my body, nothing about consent, nothing about pregnancy."

"I fully thought cis men could pee out of their butts during sex so that they didn't accidentally pee in a vagina and I didn't realize how stupid that is until I was like eighteen."

"Boys' sex drives are like a high-speed train: hard to stop once they get going. Girls' sex drives are like a cute little bicycle: not that hard to stop and not very fast. It's the girl's job to make sure the sex drives don't take them all the way to sex."

"That 'homosexuals' had short, disease-ridden lives, marked by shame, pain, loneliness, and mental illness."

"First-time sex should be painful and female orgasms are somehow elusive, rare, or difficult to achieve."

"You're supposed to put the dental dam at the back of your mouth before performing fellatio."

"If I masturbate I'll go blind."

CULPRIT 3: PURITY CULTURE

I was a beautiful child but an ugly adolescent. Acne ravaged my body years before my friends' armpits smelled, and my dry-yet-somehow-greasy curls landed in an equilateral triangle above my shoulders, something I was quick to point out, lest somebody else beat me to it. I was well-liked but not desired; socially fine but not popular. Constant, exacting performances carried me well through middle school, a chaotic home life, and beyond. At the end of school lunch, for attention, I'd goad my friends into betting their pocket change that I couldn't eat the leftover tuna salad sandwich in the middle of the table, pushed away by someone who'd deemed it inedible. I would perform eating it, theatrically, relishing the visibility. It got laughs. Did I mention I wasn't beautiful?

One day at lunch, a day I didn't binge-eat old tuna, my friend recounted a date at the movies with the boy who was now her boyfriend, in the middle school sense of the word. At the movies they had made out: French-kissed, to be exact. I tried to catch every single word without showing too much enthusiasm, which might betray my naiveté. The idea of French kissing was shocking to me. We were children! And yet I was envious, even of the casual way she said that his mouth tasted like Cheetos, like it was no big deal, and that he felt her boobs. I feared and loved the way she criticized his big, open-mouth kissing, that my friend was in a position to discern good kissing from bad kissing, while I wondered if anyone would ever like me back. After lunch, I lingered with another friend, still processing that someone in my social circle had done kissing. Decades later, I am still haunted by something I said during this debrief: "At this rate, she's going to be the first one to lose her virginity." My tone wasn't malicious, but in my mental retelling I hear a tinge of judgment, of wide-eyed astonishment that had me assessing how "fast" she was. I had already caught sex anxiety, but how? I didn't go to church, I watched mainly *SpongeBob,* and my sex ed so far had just been periods and wet dreams. The deftness with which purity culture and its main talking points—the idea that virginity is something precious to take or *lose*—shape young minds is haunting, and it haunts me today, that it got to me like that, despite my aggressively secular upbringing. *At this rate, she's going to be the first one to lose her virginity.* Why did that feel so noteworthy? I basically didn't even know what balls were. But I knew sex was trouble.

Despite growing up in a fairly progressive household, I never got a sex talk. Like many millennials, my exposure to the concept of puberty was *The Care and Keeping of You,* an illustrated American Girl book that appeared in my house one day with no explanation. (I'll never forget the relief I felt reading the page that said it was okay for breasts to be different shapes.)

Most of us learn about sex accidentally. In first grade, a class-mate asked me if I wanted to know what sex was, I said please no, she said it's when a boy puts his penis in a girl's vagina, and I told her to leave me alone. Increasingly, pop culture is reaching us faster and earlier than out-of-line classmates, teaching us about sex through our screens. "At this rate, she's going to be the first one to lose her virginity." Where did I learn that?

Traditional Puritan-Protestant values continue to implic-itly influence the judgments, behaviors, and moral cognition of contemporary Americans—not only among the devout, but also less religious Americans.[14] This has seeped into classrooms: the emphasis on sex within marriage and condemnation of pro-miscuity are two primary characteristics of what is commonly referred to as "purity culture," or the contemporary evangelical movement to promote abstinence prior to marriage, that has in-filtrated society at large, most notably in sex education. Young women are taught that they are responsible not only for their purity, but for that of the men who want to have sex with them, because they cannot help it.

Culture writer Char Adams, who is cis and straight, was raised in a conservative Christian household in Philadelphia. The first lessons she learned about sex were terrifying, she re-calls, the main one being: if you have sex before marriage, you are bad and going to hell. When she had her first kiss at thir-teen, she spiraled into a deep depression.

"I shared a part of my body, and so now I'm bad and dirty and going to hell," she remembered thinking. "That was the crux of my sex education: it's for people who were married, adult, and not gay."

At the time, the consequences of the kiss felt permanent and devastating. "A teaching that is extremely popular among Black Christians is that when you have sex, a part of that person lives in your body forever," she told me. "[So] later, if you ever experience anything like anxiety or depression, your mind quickly goes, 'Oh, it's because he's still in me.' That person's soul is now tied to yours and you can't ever get free of it."

Adams suspects that many of these teachings, even after she refuted them, lived on in her body, the way we now know that trauma does. She became sexually active at twenty, but stopped having sex when she was twenty-two, falling into a four-year celibacy. She had realized that even after intellectually unlearning some of the more toxic teachings of the church, she couldn't fully shake its influence. She hadn't been having sex that felt safe, fair, and pleasurable.

"No matter how long you unlearn these things or make choices to live differently, the messages that we get around sex and pleasure from the moment we are born is that sex is for men and that it is their pleasure experience," she said. "It is their wheelhouse, they are in control, and everything else is unimportant. We end up ignoring our desire for the sake of pleasing partners."

There are disruptive physical effects, too. Many women whose upbringings were steeped in purity culture report vaginismus, or a physical tightening of the vagina that makes intercourse extremely painful—the condition is often linked to fear or shame surrounding sex.[15] Dr. Marlene Well, a psychologist in San Francisco, coined the diagnosis "Religious Trauma Syndrome" to describe the cluster of PTSD-like symptoms "experienced by people who are struggling with leaving an authoritarian, dogmatic religion and coping with the damage of indoctrination," including anxiety disorders, depression, and sexual difficulty. PTSD leaves victims with several physical side effects that impair sexual functioning at every stage of intimacy, such as desire, arousal, and orgasm.[16]

"A big part of purity culture is that my pleasure, especially as a Black woman, is not important," Adams told me. "What isn't talked about when we talk about power dynamics of sex and relationships and the messages we get around them, especially for women, nonbinary folks, and trans folks, is that your pleasure and desires are secondary to a person's power when there is a power dynamic present. A lot of people are conditioned to conform to that norm."

These messages are so ingrained in American culture that you don't have to be raised in a conservative Christian household to internalize them.

My parents didn't teach me that sex was shameful, or that if I touched a penis its spirit would live inside me forever. But while I've never felt ashamed of the casual sex I've had, shame is still woven into the fabric of my sexual experiences. What is it, if not shame of pleasure, that would compel me to stop a man giving me oral sex that I was enjoying, because I was nervous about wasting his time? Because I felt frightened that he wasn't getting enough pleasure?

Adams has been struck by the pervasiveness of sexual values she once thought were confined to Christian culture. When I told her I wasn't raised religiously, she was surprised to learn that I went through many of the same struggles she did: a near paralysis when it came to feeling pleasure with a partner, and a hypervigilance toward that partner's pleasure.

I didn't need the church to teach me my pleasure mattered less than the men I fucked, even the monsters who faked putting on condoms because it was too dark to notice and I was beer-and-shot tipsy. I still cared about these people having a better time than me! The version of sex that I'd internalized throughout adolescence, when my friend told me (against my will!) that sex was a penis in a vagina, was an activity that wasn't supposed to feel good for me. The parts that I later learned were for me—oral sex, (controlled!) nipple stuff, and just a sprinkle of penis in vagina—I had to figure out on my own.

"The reason there's such a massive orgasm gap between the sexes is because we overvalue men's most common way of reaching an orgasm (intercourse) and undervalue women's most common way (clitoral stimulation)," Mintz wrote in *Becoming Cliterate*. The cultural overemphasis on penis-in-vagina sex deprives people of orgasms, as does the relegation of clitoral stimulation to pre-main-event foreplay, when for many, clitoral stimulation should be the headliner. But if you've spent your whole life absorbing the message that other people's pleasure matters more than your own, it's easy to go along with this.

Eli Sachse, the forty-one-year-old nurse from Northern California, told me, "Among my peers, people assigned female at birth, pleasure is just not something that was addressed when we were growing up. And I don't know how many friends of mine have said, 'I don't think I've ever had an orgasm but I'm not sure.' How sad is that?"

CULPRIT 4: WE'RE TOO SCARED AND
TIRED TO COMMUNICATE

I can count five or so men in my sexual history who've spent too much time on my nipples. This may not seem like a lot, given how many men you imagine I've slept with, but it sort of is: telling someone, "That's enough, thanks," should be pretty straightforward.

I never communicated to these five or so men that nipple time was too much because I am terrified of confrontation, but also because these five or so men were sensitive to criticism—a classically human trait. Therein lies the problem. Sensitivity, especially in relationships, is not uncommon; perceived slights set off chain reactions of resentment and hurt that ripple for months or years, and make sex feel even more fraught. Many young people still struggle to communicate with their partners about sex, even when they know communication is the fix.

"I know that communication is the only way to have good sex, but too often I'm drunk or otherwise at a place where I feel obligated to go along with things," a thirty-three-year-old cis straight man told me.

A thirty-four-year-old cis bi man told me he's grown reluctant to communicate his full identity with sexual partners due to past reactions. "I've found straight girls don't seem to believe bi guys exist, and when they find out I've slept with men think either I'm either secretly gay or HIV positive," he said.

Much of sex therapy tackles communication, and unpacking the emotional blocks that prevent us from speaking out before, during, and after unsatisfying sex. Yet again, we can shake our fists at society. When are we to learn about intimate communication? Certainly not in high school. Certainly not from *Gossip Girl*. And certainly not in the moment, when you are laser-focused on concealing the body part you hate most, or mustering every scrap of concentration to keep your dick hard, because you've learned sex begins and ends with your boner.

"There's a huge lack of modeling around intimate communication," Carole Cain, a sex therapist and educator, told me. "The Hollywood model is two people meet each other, they throw off their clothes, they jump on each other. They go home happy; nobody says a word. And you know, a lot of times students want to know why that's not happening to them."

"I don't go to that many movies, but nobody talks about condoms," Cain added. "Occasionally you'll see a used one on the floor, a sex scene of some kind, but there's no conversation about [it] exactly. Nobody ever says, 'This works for me and that doesn't'—people are just supposed to know, or the hormones are going to take care of it."

One thirty-year-old cis-het man put it to me like this: "Once sex is engaged, my ability to communicate through verbal means goes away almost immediately. I have no ability to say things without feeling stupid. Given that communication is so central to having good sexual experiences, that's a huge handicap."

This feeling is common. If the awkwardness doesn't get you, the lethargy will. Communicating feels like work. "I wish more guys were better at sex so that I wouldn't have to do so much work to find satisfying sex partners," a thirty-year-old cis-het woman lamented to me. "But I also do nothing in the way of instructing men on how to be better at sex, so I'm not really doing much to combat this issue."

Our understandable reticence to communicate about sex—during, before, and after—has a real impact on our sexual well-being. Couples who communicate about sex have been shown to experience greater orgasm frequency and sexual satisfaction.[17] Numerous studies have shown that frequent sexual communication is a sign of healthy long-term relationships.[18] For people in relationships where there is an imbalance in sexual desire, honest communication is the only way to work through it. Yet many of us still harbor a deep resistance to vocalizing our needs, or face negative reactions to trying.

I spoke with a thirty-year-old cis straight woman, who I'll call Sarah, who has been dating her boyfriend for several years. One night, about two years into their relationship, she told him that talking about sex was a turn-on for her, almost an extension of foreplay—saying what she liked and wanted, and hearing what her partner liked and wanted. Sarah's boyfriend was hurt and confused. *Had she been silently enduring sex she hated for two whole years?* He was distraught. So was Sarah—she had made herself vulnerable and faced complete rebuke. More than that, she was turned off sexually, even more so than she already had been; she wanted to be with someone she could fantasize with. He eventually realized he had overreacted and apologized. In the months since, he has evolved away from his view that sex must be unspoken to be passionate, and that it can never be planned or discussed or improved upon. But Sarah still harbors some resentment. They have sex about once a week, on the weekends; to her, it feels compulsory. She estimates that only a quarter of the sex satisfies her, even though she usually orgasms.

"It's a formula that we know works, so we fall back on it, and the sex ends up being boring and predictable," she told me. That's not to say it's terrible. "We feel close after, and I feel like it's good, but not because I liked it." Sarah is one of many people in relationships who tolerate so-so sex because the only two things that could change it—communication, or a breakup—feel too daunting. This hopelessness even extends to people who know the solution, and Sarah knows the solution; communication played a vital role in the success and failures of her past relationships. While her current partner has developed a willingness to talk about sex, she feels unmotivated to try again with him. It's a classic case of burnout.

"I feel like there is potential for it to be better. I would just have to put in work to get there, which is true for a lot of things in a relationship," she said. "I don't think we have the best sexual chemistry that I've ever experienced in my life. [But] in a way, it's the best sex, because it's so familiar."

The bar is low. She knows she could raise it, but she doesn't have the energy.

"I don't know how much it matters to me. It gets confusing," she said. "If you have boring sex for a long time, your libido does go down and you don't really care anymore. And it becomes kind of comfortable. It becomes less and less important over time. I feel like I could take steps to fix the problem, but my motivation level to do that fluctuates."

While this book aims to illuminate the benefits of less-bad

sex and less bad sex, it also respects the calculations we make surrounding sex, even bad sex. (Remember, bad sex is not shameful!) For Sarah, the calculation right now is: I don't have the energy. That's okay. Balancing this dialectic of acceptance and change is the only way we can maintain compassion for ourselves, a prerequisite for any personal growth, sexual or otherwise.

In an era where the internet has outsized influence in the construction of our sexual identities, much of this work happens online—for better and mostly worse.

3

CYBERSEX LIVES

NAVIGATING DIGITAL MEDIA

"Internet dating had evolved to present the world around us,
the people in our immediate vicinity, and to fulfill the desires
of a particular moment. At no point did it offer guidance in
what to do with such a vast array of possibility."

—*Emily Witt,* Future Sex

It's hard to recall how I found people to have sex with before dating apps became mainstream enough for a coward like me to download them. Periodically, I'm hit with flashbacks of standing in moist, chaotic bars in lower Manhattan, wearing skintight dresses that keep migrating above my thighs and willing moist, chaotic men to approach me. I remember one night that could have been any night: sipping a cloying vodka Red Bull, I surveyed the scene of grinding youths and exchanged notes with a cluster of girls I don't speak to anymore, not due to drama but rather limited bandwidth. (Most of them are happily married, and my hands are full with self-improvement projects.) Who was cute? Who was looking at me? Who was looking at the hotter girl behind me? These were the questions.

After an hour or so of nervous shoulder dancing, I spotted a tall man with a severe jaw, leaning on the bar with a sense of authority. He looked like he worked in consulting. Everybody looked like they worked in consulting, I felt, except me, a downtrodden writer who made crude generalizations about others to feel unique. Those days, it felt like all you had to do to initiate flirtation was simply to place yourself near someone and make an observation. "It's humid in here," I shouted, yanking my dress down. Later that night we had middling stranger sex at his sterile apartment. I kept accidentally making eye contact with the paperback copy of *The Secret* on his bedside table, so it's safe to say I didn't orgasm, but that wasn't the point. The point was for me to pass the time and feel attractive for a few moments because I struggled to do either of these things on my own. I noticed recently that we're friends on Facebook, and he is married. It's fine. I'm fine.

So beLIEVE me, I would never romanticize the days of schlepping myself to hookup bars in hopes of meeting day traders because I couldn't afford my own well drinks. In many respects, the normalization of dating apps like Hinge, Tinder, and OkCupid have upgraded my sexual experiences: I can meet people I'm more compatible with, at least on paper, and more easily filter out those with views I find reprehensible (fitness is NOT, in fact, "life"). The apps expanded my sexual options beyond just people I approached because I was wasted, and not being wasted for all my sexual experiences has done wonders for quality. For LGBTQIA+ people, who have historically had smaller pools of potential partners, the apps revolutionized dating and hooking up, making it safer, easier, and, for many people, more pleasurable, and online forums have long made dating more accessible for disabled people. Feeld, a remarkably inclusive dating app that surged during the pandemic, filled a great need for polyamorous and/or kinky people, while welcoming all kinds of daters, swingers, and casual fuckers with "alternative" sexual preferences. Progress, I dare say, is good. Generally.

There is, of course, a catch. The apps empower us all to feel like Olivia Colman in *The Favourite,* selecting the partners we find most pleasing with the fatigued swipe of a finger. Like Colman, we feel that if we just keep looking, it's possible we could connect with Emma Stone, or at least the guys I date do. (They're delusional!!) But has the dating app revolution given us better relationships? Are we having better sex? Are we more romantically fulfilled because we dodged the bullet of getting coffee with a man who holds trout in photos?

I don't have the answers to these questions. I just know I'm miserable.

Smartphones have solved many of the trickiest parts of our sex lives—finding people, screening people, allowing horny but tired people to stay in their homes while coordinating sex opportunities—but they've also complicated our experience of sex. The perception of unlimited choice has made us more anxious about finding the perfect partner or relationship, since we have more information up front, offering us the illusion of agency. This "paradox of choice," as American psychologist Barry Schwartz would call it, and infinite swiping mentality can leave us feeling more responsible for curating super fulfilling, orgasmic romantic lives, and even more disappointed when our experiences don't measure up. We (I) think that our ability to screen out Patriots fans will help us (me) find more compatible partners, but that's not necessarily true. Maybe the love of my life is a Patriots fan and I will never know because these apps empower me to block and report them with a tap of the thumb. We feel like we have unlimited options, the people we have sex with feel like they have unlimited options, and we are all anxious about it.

These conditions have created a new class of lousy sexual prospects that I like to call The Ones Who Never Got Away. I remember when Frank Ocean's *Blonde* dropped in 2016, listening to it in Bushwick Inlet Park, on the jumbo rocks that line the East River. My phone lit up; someone I'd slept with four years ago had liked my tweet—our first communication in four years. A month before that, a different man from my past, who I'll call Brad, commented on a dog-filtered selfie I'd posted on Snapchat: "10/10." Brad, who I'd never had sex with or even met in person, had been lurking on the fringes of my life for over three years, after we'd matched on Tinder and talked briefly. The conversation had come to a screeching halt after he texted me footage of his penis ejaculating, unprompted. But that summer of *Blonde,* years later, this man was still around, even if virtually, even though I'd never met him and/or seen his non-dick parts. I didn't know why or how I was still connected to him on any social media platform; I remembered unfriending him on Facebook and blocking him on Instagram. Brad is one of The Ones Who Never Got Away.

While I never ended up sleeping with Brad, I've slept with plenty of Ones Who Never Got Away years after things "ended." Most people dating today have a similar cast of characters— people who keep popping up in their lives, people who never go away. They stay, and they stay, and they stay, because where there is a 1 percent chance of something happening, there is staying. Staying looks like heart-ing an Instagram from sixty-three weeks ago, like texting "you in the city?" to someone you matched with years ago but never actually met. Staying is so easy.

The prospect of closing off a romantic opportunity—or looking like you care enough to delete, block, or unfollow—can feel so daunting that I somehow stayed Snapchat friends with gross Brad. The phenomenon of sloppy endings is not new. But the phenomenon of people enduring and enduring—people who've been gifted the shelf life of freeze-dried astronaut snacks—*is*. This contemporary technological hellscape has made it possible to collect people you can never quite lose, contributing to a frenzied climate of infinite sexual possibilities and infinite ways to burn out. Too often, we go back to them when we're at our lowest, desperate for connection we aren't getting elsewhere.

In addition to deftly storing people from our past, people we would do well to forget, smartphones have also exposed us to more harassment, more losers, and more indignities, like discovering our ex has redownloaded Tinder, even though he said he "needed a breather from dating." However, while dating app culture has created new problems, it cannot be blamed for all the bad sex we have. The apps have made it *easier* to have bad sex, but only because they made it easier to have sex at all.

I am glad dating apps exist. I'm too tired to go to bars, let alone go to bars with an agenda. It is not Hinge's fault that, during a recent three-minute stretch of oral sex, I wondered if the charming throw blanket I'd seen on the Anthropologie website would go on sale soon, nor is it responsible for the other things that make sex hard to enjoy, like the body-shaming, slut-shaming, and general sex negativity that more screen time forces us to digest more of. While writing this chapter and generally minding my own business, the Instagram algorithm served me a video of a Bible influencer dancing behind text that read, "When you realize the 'independent woman' role culture sold you was negatively impacting God's design for your marriage." (This same influencer, who instructs on how to "protect your purity" while married, also makes cutesy videos about why you shouldn't have friends of the opposite sex if you want to preserve "emotional oneness" with your husband.) It's clear to me that the primary sexual saboteur is not dating apps but apps at large, and their near-total monopolization of our attention, even in the (rare) instances we're not scrolling.

To be clear, moralizing around technology is my nightmare. I refuse to idealize decades past, where we may have been more ~*present*~ in the absence of smartphones but also sanitary pads came with belts and every marginalized group had fewer rights.

The positive impacts of technology and, more specifically, the internet, on quality of life are innumerable. Social media networks foster community-building and information-disseminating that couldn't happen otherwise. Given the heteronormative horrors of contemporary sexual education, the internet is the only safe place for many people to access medically accurate, trans-inclusive information about sexual health. For young queer people who cannot safely come out, social media offers what can be lifesaving community. On a neurological level, studies have shown that the connections we make on social media are processed just like the ones we make in the offline world, and "carry over from the internet to shape 'real-world' sociality."[1]

What is relatively new, and ominous, is technology's capacity to rewire our brains, including the neural pathways where we seek and process pleasure. The apps that populate our smartphones are modeled after slot machines, in order to best monopolize (and commodify) our attention, making it harder for us to appreciate slower, less-immediate pleasures in the offline world.[2] Anyone who has ever tried to read a book, only to reflexively check Twitter every three minutes, can recognize that smartphones have eroded our attention spans. For most of us, who need time and buildup to experience sexual pleasure, this is bad news: If we require fifteen to twenty minutes of clitoral stimulation to reach orgasm, but have an attention span of three to five, sexual satisfaction will remain out of reach, no matter how skilled our partners, no matter how expensive our sex toys, no matter how vocal our sex-positivity.

"It's a pace issue," *Pleasure Activism* author adrienne maree brown told me. "We're moving in a world where every single thing that is happening is urgent. Feeling contentment and satisfaction is actually often tied to stepping out of the urgency."

Recent studies show that increased smartphone usage is linked to decreased capacity to feel pleasure in the body.[3] (Oh hey, anhedonia!) On a neurobiological level, technology addiction functions just like any other, offering dopamine hits that we start to crave all the time. People with addictive social media habits—i.e., most of us, because apps are designed to be addictive—become "unable to experience the natural 'high' of positive feelings from a release of dopamine triggered by the experience of everyday living," [4] writes Dr. Wise in *Why Good Sex Matters*. "They get caught in a loop of seeking more and more and more, which often leads to escalating compulsive behaviors." Our bodies are hardwired to seek pleasure for our survival—in the form of food, sex, and safety, for example—so when this process is interrupted by a never-ending barrage of notifications, we become saddled with dissatisfaction: always seeking more but increasingly feeling less.

"Our technology-driven, constantly connected culture reinforces this disruption of our pleasure system," Wise writes. "Television binge-watching, nonstop texting, Snapchats, checking Instagram, and other repetitive behaviors that now happen almost automatically keep us distracted and numb, hijacking our neural pathways at critical points." As Wise points out, tech engineers design their products with the express purpose of keeping us hooked—and dissatisfied. When we are stuck in this loop of perpetual seeking, "we enter a state of 'pleasure shutdown,' never quite getting the opportunity to learn to feel our pleasure more fully, to savor the sensations."

Beyond the erosion of our ability to concentrate, experience contentment, and stay present, our saturation in digital media can engender toxic thought patterns that distort our sexual experiences. This brings us to problem number two: not only do digital platforms affect the way we experience the world by virtue of their design, but the actual content on those platforms wield ever-increasing power over us. One particularly vulnerable demographic is teen girls; Facebook's own research found that Instagram has a significant negative impact on their mental health and self-image.[5]

Our little screens perpetuate shame, misinformation, and unrealistic expectations for sex, dating, and intimacy, most notably via porn and social media.[6] Idealized, unattainable depictions of sex and romance are not new—as a child, I yearned for what Julia Roberts and Richard Gere have in *Runaway Bride*—but the current *scale* of these depictions is unprecedented. We are constantly getting pummeled with normative fantasies on an ever-multiplying number of platforms, rendering those fantasies more powerful and dangerous. To orient you: in 1970, the average American child began watching television regularly at age four. A recent study found that kids began interacting with digital media, on average, at four months.[7]

The process of internalizing sexual norms begins in childhood, during small moments—of getting yelled at for grinding on a pillow, unknowingly masturbating; of watching movie couples orgasm in sync; of hearing gay slurs on the playground. Our understanding of what sexuality can and should be incubates in our soft kid brains long before we start having sex and even longer before we find ourselves wholeheartedly accepting that sex with our fiancé will never feel great but that he offers other things, like bringing home wine sometimes. The way "good sex" is modeled to us via digital media, like porn and movies—cis-heterosexual penis-vagina sex where the woman is awash in pleasure despite zero clitoral stimulation—is bad sex for most people with vulvas, who are unable to orgasm from penetration alone. And then there's the extreme, outcome-centric emphasis on erection and penile orgasm—to signal the beginning and end of sex, respectively—that creates undue anxiety and pressure to perform. "Given that in most situations, at least in my experience, I'm running the show, if it's bad, it's probably my fault," one thirty-year-old cis-het man told me.

Unlearning reductive, patriarchal sexual norms requires education, exploration, and—because we are dealing with humans—communication. When we are failed by education, exploration and communication become more challenging. We don't know how to communicate. We're scared; we're tired. Our vocabulary for communicating during sex is deeply limited, and when we believe our pleasure matters less, why speak up?

Purity culture and cis-heteronormativity pervade popular culture so profoundly that it actually disrupts our sexual development. Messages about what sex is and isn't live in our bodies long after we believe we've unlearned them—messages like "There's something wrong with me if I can't orgasm during penetrative sex," "My job during sex is to make my partner orgasm," and "I'm a bad, horrible slut for sleeping with so many people." Even Emily Ratajkowski, a model and author who is arguably one of the hottest people on the planet, is not immune, admitting in a recent TikTok, "Women have internalized the male gaze so much, that when we're having sex, we're thinking about how hot or not we are." These preoccupations aren't always tethered to specific thoughts, but they can disrupt us before, during, and after sex with unpleasant body sensations, sensations that feel a lot like shame, anxiety, and numbness. Like trauma responses, these sensations bubble up when we least expect it, making it even harder for us to feel pleasure and enjoy sex. Bad sex becomes the norm.

Through popular culture, we internalize expectations for sex that spoil it for us. *Bridgerton,* the steamy Netflix period drama from Shonda Rhimes, promised to be different, progressive. Set in the Regency period of England, the show chronicles the scandalous goings-on of London's elite during courting season. Rhimes's modern sensibility and proven track record of strong female characters (*Scandal, Grey's Anatomy*) suggested to me that the period lovemaking would also be a breath of fresh air. And in many ways, it was. We see a woman masturbating! We see cunnilingus!

But as much as the show liberated itself from the confines of historical accuracy, the sex was disappointingly old-fashioned. When protagonist Daphne Bridgerton has sex for the first time, she and the Duke of Hastings orgasm at the same time . . . from penetrative sex. In fact, during most of the sex scenes, they orgasm at the same time . . . from penetrative sex alone . . . when over 80 percent of women can never reach orgasm from penetrative sex alone. Maybe Daphne Bridgerton is a sex prodigy, but I'm sorry, this is fucked. Why can't we see them have exhilarating, passionate sex where she or he doesn't come? *Bridgerton* is a fantasy, yes, but fantasies have power; they shape our desire— and can set us up for disappointment. I'm tired of every pop culture fantasy priming us to feel shitty about the sex that is most accessible to us.

Author and sex educator Gabrielle Alexa Noel came out as bisexual after years of dating men. The society-wide minimization

of clitoral stimulation makes perfect sense to her. The pop culture we consume is born of the patriarchy, which says again
and again: sex is for men with dicks. The real-world impact of
this messaging is that penetrative sex feels compulsory, which
enforces imbalances in pleasure, and even harms the men who
supposedly benefit from it.

"In the absence of sex education, unfortunately, as much as
I blame the patriarchy, what do we expect from men who are
also people and aren't informed about vulvas?" Noel told me.
"They learn and internalize that sex is penetration, and the only
type of sex that's spoken about in sex education is penetration,
and that other sexual behaviors that should just count as sex
are relegated to foreplay, which makes it seem almost optional.
When it seems like a precursor to sex, then it becomes something that people rush through, even though I think a lot of
people with vulvas need lengthy foreplay, or even only want
what's described as foreplay."

Noel always knew foreplay was important while dating
men, but when she began dating women, she struggled to unlearn this idea that penetration was "full" sex. "That was deeply
freeing," she said. "I think a lot of straight people would benefit
from knowing that, because they feel fucking crazy when they
think penetration is just whatever."

≈ ≈

There is no escape from "false images"—that is, images that
feel authentic but are produced, constructed, political. The images we're exposed to about sex and our bodies, specifically—

especially during our adolescence—are uniquely harmful. At no point in history have we been more aware of how we are supposed to look, what we are supposed to do, and who we are supposed to be—in large part thanks to the internet. During the Italian Renaissance, the ideal female form was a pasty-skinned woman with big breasts, round stomach, and full hips. Let's say you did not look like that: your skin had pigmentation, your breasts were little nubs, and your stomach was flat, no matter how much spaghetti you ate to bulk up. There would certainly be moments in daily life where you'd be reminded that your body did not meet contemporary beauty standards; perhaps you had fewer romantic prospects, or your nonna made disparaging comments. Maybe, if you were of a certain stature, you visited museums and gazed upon paintings that glorified the rotund women you so desperately yearned to resemble. But, for the most part, you lived your life, occupying yourself with more pressing concerns. The streets flowed with sewage!

Today, if a person has even one body part that deviates from prevailing beauty standards, they will be reminded of it every minute or so: scrolling TikTok on the toilet, deep-diving Olivia Rodrigo's Instagram while waiting in line for coffee, opening a magazine, watching a movie, passing an ad on a bus, passing an ad on a billboard, watching porn on the bus while passing an ad on a billboard. The pace is dizzying: in the time it took me to write that paragraph, the Kardashian women reportedly took out their BBLs, and we as a nation must scramble to adapt. (A violently toxic *New York Post* headline has declared that "Heroin chic is back," as though we might want to take cues.)[8]

We'll return to social media, but most of these false images are relayed through pornography. A thirty-seven-year-old cis straight man, who I'll call Henry, told me that he is still grappling with his early exposure to porn, which he had no tools to make sense of at the time. He felt he became addicted to it around age thirteen, as he attempted to dissociate from a turbulent home life and figure out his own sexuality. "Porn started to shape my expectations such that, as a thirteen-year-old male with access to this new technology 'AIM,' I felt pressured to find a girl to have sex with," Henry said. (For the infants reading this, AIM stands for AOL Instant Messenger. Think of it as TikTok DMs of the olden days.) "I remember how awful that felt. It also led to older men and women contacting me." Porn was his sexual education, as it is for many American adolescents. There is nothing inherently nefarious about porn, but it is performance. And when children aren't taught the difference between real sex and performance sex, it can lead to dissatisfaction in their sex lives for years to come.[9] One cis straight man in his thirties told me that his early exposure to violent hardcore porn gave him unrealistic expectations for what sex would be: he learned from porn, for example, that it's hot to choke your partner without asking. While he has since learned to get consent before strangling someone, he is still most turned on by sex that emulates the porn he grew up with, and he feels a lot of shame about it.

Somehow I never sought out porn as an adolescent; maybe I was too busy cleaning up pixelated vomit on the streets of *Roller-Coaster Tycoon*. My AIM experience was painfully unsexual, too. I chatted with friends occasionally, but I was far more interested in crafting away messages that underscored just how misunderstood I was: *"Don't criticize what you don't understand"—bob dylan. xoxo.* It's also likely that our family computer's very public placement on top of the staircase de-incentivized any impulse to seek cybersex or ask Jeeves what semen was. While I didn't personally find porn, I did devour a 2004 issue of *Us Weekly* with Jessica Simpson on the cover, entitled, "How I Keep Nick Happy," one of many cues I internalized in my most formative years that taught me healthy relationships resemble a sort of servitude.

When it comes to porn, I recognize that I'm in the minority; porn exposure and online sexual activity reaches adolescents earlier (now around eleven) and more easily (literally anywhere) than ever. This isn't as dangerous as news anchors might have you believe, but there are long-lasting consequences when exposure to sexualized images is not coupled with media literacy. Sex education's failure to acknowledge that kids are horny online is a massive policy failure with moral implications: those horny kids become adults who still struggle to navigate their sexual lives.

"Pornography is not sex education, and it should never be looked at that way . . . and I don't think the onus of responsibility is on us to educate the public," said Jacky St. James, a pornography writer and director, in a 2019 NPR feature on the impact of porn. "I think that should be done in the school system and with parents, but certainly it's not our responsibility. And I don't think a lot of people are willing to accept that. They want to blame us for everything, and I'm not going to be blamed, because it's a fantasy—that's what we're creating at the end of the day." [10]

Wherever you place the blame, the problem remains that fantasies impact our realities. In that same NPR feature, a twenty-six-year-old college student recounted what it was like to have sex for the first time after years of watching porn. It hadn't even dawned on him that the porn was fantasy, not a true-to-life portrayal, until he became sexually active. He was shocked, for example, that his first sexual experience didn't last for an hour and a half. A twenty-three-year-old woman named Danielle said, "I don't really know if my boyfriend has watched porn or not, but I feel like he has brought expectations into the relationship, and sometimes I feel bad because I can't meet those expectations, so I feel like something's wrong with me."

Studies show that adolescents' exposure to porn shapes their attitudes toward gender, sexuality, and relationships well into adulthood. One study (of largely white, largely heterosexual men) found the average age of porn exposure to be 13.3, with the youngest being 5 and the oldest being 26. The younger the male was exposed to porn, "the more likely he was to want power over women later on." The later the exposure, "the more likely he would want to engage in playboy behavior." [11] Playboy behavior, here, is defined as being sexually promiscuous. There's a lot to dislike about this study, namely the homogeneity among participants and the gendering of promiscuity, but it helpfully illuminates the power of porn to shape behavior. Of course, there is nothing wrong with sexual promiscuity (I engage in playboy behavior myself), but when we let expectations override our genuine desires, we're disappointed. We remain unsatisfied.

"I think it's lazy when we blame porn entirely for what people are into, when it's a reflection of patriarchy and racism and all of those other isms and phobias," Noel told me. "But, it still feeds it in many ways when you're only seeing people enjoy pleasure who look a certain way. It almost feels like a message that gets internalized, that you don't deserve it." Noel said she is careful to be intentional about her porn consumption.

"I push myself to consume content that involves people of color, because I feel like otherwise the translation in my body, regardless of my personal narrative, is that I start to question my own identity and how people are perceiving the attractiveness of me as a Black woman," she said. "I'm very intentional about seeking movies and TV in general. I make sure that I consume a lot of content that has people of color, so I'm always providing myself with the additional representation that normative society is erasing."

One thirty-one-year-old cis gay man I spoke with, who I'll call Bill, discovered porn in third grade by googling "boobs." He credits porn with helping him figure out his sexuality. With no gay people in his family and actively homophobic friends, he said it may not have occurred to him that he was gay had he not found gay porn—it was his only exposure to other people like him. "I accidentally stumbled upon gay porn in middle school and my reaction was to be like, 'That's terrible.' And then I thought, maybe not," he said. "Porn helped me figure out my sexuality faster than I would have. But it didn't help me come to terms with it faster."

Bill recalls feeling insecure about the ripped, chiseled porn stars, who taught him that a "hot" body didn't look anything like his. He eventually got over that, and now easily separates the fantasy of porn from the kind of sex he actually likes ("in real life I gravitate toward more realistic bodies.") But the fact remains that porn was his sexual education. "It's very difficult imagining a world without porn," he said. "How would I even know about things?"

Social media is another powerful vessel for "false images"—images, like Bill's ripped, chiseled porn stars—that tell us we are unworthy of pleasure, that other people are having better and more sex, that our desires are weird or wrong.

Increasingly, our sexualities develop in conversation with social media. Regardless of our upbringings, we internalize the norms and taboos that populate our feeds, which shape the way we see the world and ourselves. Scholars of gender have suggested that social media pushes us to perform gender and sexual identity as "coherent, stable, and fixed entities," preventing us from "being open to the dynamic and diverse ways genders and sexual identities are lived in everyday life."[12] This pressure to perform extends beyond gender and sexual identity: whether we're posting thirst traps or highlight reels of romantic relationships, we are performing the versions of our identities most likely to elicit likes—a dynamic that can further cement the disconnect from our truest, most authentic sexual selves. "We're always driven by and reacting to external stimuli—others' needs, others' perceptions—and social media is a cesspool where all of that is at the forefront," Hailey Magee, a life coach who specializes in codependency, told me. "We developed a disconnected relationship from ourselves."

This obsession with external stimuli is fostered on dating apps, as well—a place where it's so easy to measure your worth in number of matches. Dating apps basically function as social media, and vice versa. In both spaces, we contort our identities to be attractive, cool, or interesting to others. At that sticky Manhattan bar all those years ago, such contortion simply wasn't an option. When I approached that consultant bro, I was wearing makeup and a slutty dress, and, sure, self-styling can be performance in its way. (The real top of my lips landed a centimeter lower than painted.) But ultimately I couldn't approach him in the way that dating apps let me approach people: with a look book of my hottest selves and my sharpest observational comedy. Furthermore, there wouldn't have even been An Approaching had the transaction been performed online. I'm certain I would have spotted a red flag and swiped on by.

On social media, or any communal platform, certain performances are rewarded more than others. Here's a high-profile example: in February 2021, Kendall Jenner posted a photo of herself inside a Barbie box, modeling her sister Kim Kardashian's new line of red Skims. (If you don't know what Skims are, it's direct-to-consumer underwear for changing the shape of your body.) Jenner posted a gleaming full-body selfie in a small red bikini top and even smaller red thong bottom; the front panel of the thong, traditionally tasked with hiding the labia, was a square no larger than an unfolded Starburst wrapper. While most people have some discoloration or razor burn or, how to put it, textural complexities around their pelvic region, Jenner's appeared to be Photoshopped into oblivion—it was sleek, smooth, symmetrical nothingness, all in one shade of Barbie doll. As of this writing, the post has 13.1 million likes.

I am mostly at peace with my quirky vulva. But seeing Jenner's lack of one, even in an image I could immediately recognize as digitally altered, made me feel bad about mine. Now imagine you are one of those 13.1 million likers who does not have a disturbingly precise understanding of photo editing, and who has not seen countless goofy-looking, asymmetrical vulvas, and who is maybe on the younger side. It may make you hate your body more than you already did. To be clear, it is not Kendall Jenner's job to teach us about how vulvas look, just like it is not porn's job to teach us about sex, but the reality is they end up doing both jobs. That leaves us with two choices: figure out a way to arm youth with tools for navigating digital content, or abandon them.

Like a growing number of social media–wary humans, adrienne maree brown has set limits. When I spoke with the *Pleasure Activism* author over the phone on a sunny spring afternoon, she said she was down to forty-five minutes a day, spread out over all her social media, including Instagram, Twitter, Facebook, and TikTok. For brown, the impact of less scrolling had been extreme and immediate. She felt changes in her body, in her attention span, "in every aspect" of her existence.

"I feel like I'm having more original ideas, and I'm able to notice more often when I am satisfied in the moment," she said. "I took a bath yesterday, and I was like, 'This bath is really excellent. I really appreciate this quality of light. And I like being able to read in this space.'"

She feels more present in every area of her life since limiting social media use. "In intimate acts, in periods of sitting and trying to be present in a conversation, I can feel a tangible difference in the quality of my attention," she said. "The scroll-ing process makes you like, 'I'm here, but my mind is always leaping ahead to the next experience, the next thing. And I'm never fully present, whatever the thing is, just leaping, leaping, leaping.' Trying to have an intimate conversation with someone whose mind is partially looking ahead at where else they're go-ing to go, or what else is happening, it can be very frustrating and hard."

If you're interested in crafting a digital life that prioritizes your sexual well-being, these tips can help loosen the grip of the internet on your brain (and make your baths more enjoyable).

~* A FEW RULES FOR HEALTHY INTERNET USE THAT CAN IMPROVE YOUR SEX LIFE *~

1. **Set screen time limits and stick to them.** I know, I know. Everybody says this and it's always annoying. But limit-ing the amount of time spent scrolling, browsing, and swiping is like a massage for your brain, and makes it easier for you to stay present in the moment (like during cunnilingus!) rather than "spectatoring." There are tons of free apps that can help you limit screen time, like BreakFree and ZenScreen, by target-ing specific apps that you know are problems for you.

"If I'm scrolling through social media for six hours a day, I'm avoiding being alone with myself," Magee, the life coach, told me. "We're so unaccustomed to spending time alone with ourselves and looking inward and being generative as opposed to reactive and being like, 'What do I really want? What am I really feeling right now?'" Physically limiting social media time allows us to process the feelings and sensations (like yearning, depression, horniness, and loneliness) that get dulled by scrolling—some of the same feelings and sensations that can shape our sex lives.

2. **Be thoughtful about the porn you consume.** Like all media, porn shapes how we experience the world and our bodies, and it can color our expectations of sex. Seek out ethically made, feminist porn—ideally porn that puts dollars directly into the pockets of sex workers—that shows all bodies are worthy of pleasure. Think beyond porn that centers cis, able-bodied, heteronormative sex, or porn that reinforces norms that don't serve you. "Most people get their sex education from porn; that's a fact that we can't divorce ourselves from," said the author and sex educator Gabrielle Alexa Noel. "When it comes to perception of who is and isn't sexy, I think porn can collaboratively participate in that." Consider spending money on independently made porn that supports creators directly, or choose a few OnlyFans accounts to support every month.

3. **Remain curious and critical of dating apps, social media, and the internet in general.** Noel's book, *How to Live with the Internet and Not Let It Run Your Life,* is a great primer for becoming an informed, critical consumer of the internet, which can help protect your self-image and mental health. Digital media has the potential to positively shape sexual culture, if we remain critical consumers; people can access information about sexual health and build affirming communities on social media platforms. "These platforms can strengthen ideas around the rigidness of sexual orientation by encouraging us to display

our orientation labels and to organize ourselves around them," writes Noel. "But they also make it more acceptable to identify as someone who isn't heterosexual."

4. **Follow sex-positive, LGBTQIA+-friendly sex educators.** Not only will this make you more comfortable thinking and talking about sex, but you will likely learn very useful things about sexual wellness that you certainly didn't learn in school, thanks to sex-positive influencers and educators. Also: unfollow people who make you feel horrible about yourself.

5. **Detox when possible.** Even if you can't take a complete break from your smartphone, see if you can take weeklong breaks (or longer!) away from dating and social media apps that are causing you more anxiety than joy. It is as natural as the cycles of the moon to delete and redownload dating apps. When evaluating aspects of your digital media consumption that feel unhealthy, you needn't take an abstinence-only approach; it's unrealistic and will make you feel bad when you inevitably open Instagram on Safari as a workaround. Give yourself grace.

4

THE POWER OF SEX CLEANSES, DRY SPELLS, AND AVOIDING SEX ALTOGETHER

"I didn't have sex for a full year and a half between 2017 and 2018. And I was so happy. I didn't shave my legs, or my whole body really, I was just satisfied with work and roller derby and my friends. I was truly fulfilled and happy without sex."
—*thirty-one-year-old cis bi woman*

To recap: sex is bad a lot. The badness of sex often stems from the ritual neglect of our own desires and sensations, because that's how we've been socialized. We feel bad about this badness because popular media has convinced us that everyone is having more and better sex than we are, and that synchronized orgasm is standard after seven seconds of penis-in-hole intercourse. We are burned out—on sex and everything else—and we don't even care that much, because how could we, when the world is crumbling down around us? Anhedonia, the clinical inability to experience pleasure, is on the rise. The media is oversexed yet we are over sex. We've refused to take the recycling out for weeks because we cannot bear the thought of doing an activity.

If this all rings depressing to you, that's because it is. There are, however, glimmers of hope. One glimmer is the growing number of sex psychologists, coaches, and educators emerging in the relatively new field of sex therapy. This is fantastic news for people with the cash to outsource sexual problem-solving, and still pretty good news for the rest of us: many of the tools and exercises used in sessions are seeping into the popular consciousness—at a glacial pace, but a pace nonetheless. In 2019, for example, *Teen Vogue* published an in-depth guide to anal sex and the requisite preparations. The only sex-adjacent awareness-building I recall from the magazines of my girlhood is just page after page of humiliating reader-submitted stories about periods—girls getting their period on their crush's back during a flirty piggyback ride, girls getting their period during gym class (swim unit), girls getting their period on their crush's back during gym class (swim unit).

My aim for this book is to illuminate some of the more promising practices within the field of sex therapy that help treat, or at least investigate, sexual dissatisfaction, both within relationships and outside of them. One tool that is near and dear to my heart? Taking sex off the table entirely. Given that so many of us are sex-recessing already, why don't we congratulate ourselves for what we were already doing?

To consciously sex-recess, we need to understand why we're having sex in the first place. A couple years after returning from Croatia, and for years, I slept with a male acquaintance quarterly, even though he was rude to me and the sex was obnoxious: he choked without asking (a theme) and kissed like a vacuum. I had vowed to stop, but how could I when I didn't understand why I was doing it? I knew our irregular, emotionally confusing hookups would lead to nothing, and I wanted *something*—but what? The hooking up felt okay in the moment, dreamy right after (were we together??), and then terrible after the right after. When enough time passed after the terrible, I would reactivate the cycle, my memory effectively wiped.

His hands couldn't do anything mine couldn't, and the psychological cost of liking him more than he liked me was greater than the fleeting coziness I felt when he initiated a spoon or reacted 🔥 on an Instagram Story. Why was I enduring this? I sat with the uneasy question until I landed on an answer: I wanted to be held. I didn't want a relationship, but I was horny for companionship. That's it. Seeking out sex that I knew would be lackluster had become an ineffectual coping mechanism that, while not actively destructive, concealed the truth of what I was feeling and what I needed, rendering it perpetually out of reach. And while there's nothing wrong with seeking sex for reasons beyond the pursuit of sexual bliss, mindfulness of my *actual* pursuit was key: I realized that no sex with him would mean better sex for me, overall. I could free up space for other ways to feel held, touched, and cared for—by myself, by friends, even by weighted blankets. And so, I began sex-recessing, on a micro scale. I scaled back on dating out of boredom. I scaled back on texting people for the sole purpose of preserving this sense of sexual chaos I'd grown so accustomed to.

Years later, I scaled back from sex entirely, for about a year.

It was the best decision I've made for my mental health in recent memory (if we don't include buying my dog little outfits). It also made sex more enjoyable when I started having it again. Of course, the decision to step back from sex was influenced by the global pandemic, which steepened emotional and physical barriers to dating—the one thing that could lead to sex for a homebound recluse like myself. I could barely coordinate seeing close friends in a way that felt safe, let alone organizing a meetup with a potential sex partner. I unwittingly slipped into the kind of sex hiatus that sex therapists often recommend to people experiencing sexual dissatisfaction. And you can, too.

Sure, in a fantasy world where Stanley Tucci is all of our husbands, we could aspire to more *and* better sex, but for now, in a world where sex can go very wrong and Stanley Tucci doesn't know we exist, our surest path is less but better sex. First and foremost: having less sex instantly ensures you are having less bad sex. That's just mathematics. You're freeing up time for other activities that offer a higher return on investment, like masturbating, reading, and cleaning that space between your bed and the wall. But the most powerful part of having less sex is that you're more inclined to hold out for sex that you love.

Janet Brito, the sex therapist in Hawaii, finds there to be enormous benefits to having less sex: you can more easily focus on developing a loving, sexual relationship with yourself and your body, "as the focus is more on the individual and less on someone else." She continued listing perks to me, including "less pressure to perform, less risk of acquiring a sexually transmitted infection, helps you to prioritize self-care and explore other ways to experience pleasure, and increased time to explore one's beliefs and attitudes about sex."

Taking a break from sex to feel better about sex makes some amount of intuitive sense: the most immediate way to stop having bad sex is to have no sex at all. But the practice is also constructive and affirming, beyond just negating the bad.

"If you're having unsatisfying sex, you may need to step back a little and see what's going on," Julia Bartz, the psychotherapist in New York, told me. "You may be feeling burnt out, or uncomfortable in your body, or too focused on your partner's pleasure at the expense of your own. You may not have spent the time or energy even figuring out what makes you feel pleasure, apart from any partners."

If sex with partners is regularly dissatisfying, exploring pleasure without a partner is the first place to troubleshoot. "Starting from square one—*What gives me pleasure?*—is the first step to bringing awareness down from the brain into the body," said Bartz. "It doesn't even have to be sexual. Maybe it's delicious food, or dancing, or taking a long walk in a park. People are often so numbed out these days that they need to teach themselves how to be sensual, or experience the world through their senses."

Intentional "dry spells"—or even those you're trapped in against your will—facilitate this kind of personal pleasure exploration that can eventually enrich partnered sexual experiences.

❧ ❧

If having sex is fraught, then so is not having it. For thousands of years, preeminent thinkers, religious figures, and medicine-adjacent philosophers have espoused the virtues of abstinence, for reasons as varied and deranged as sex itself. In fact, the directive to abstain from sex for a given length of time existed long before we suspected that God wanted us to do so, and that sexual activity was a barometer of purity and goodness.

Galen, the Roman philosopher and physician of the second century, is featured prominently in the third edition of Foucault's groundbreaking work *History of Sexuality.* At the turn of the millennium, the pathologizing of sex gained real steam, laying the framework for the very sex anxiety we know and hate today. While thinkers at the time suspected that sex had the capacity to heal—for example, some believed semen to be a type of phlegm, and that expelling it could alleviate respiratory illnesses—they warned of the harm sex could cause if the subject was in poor condition. Galen wrote that people who ejaculate too much, for example, "experience a languor at the stomach orifice, exhaustion, weakness, and dryness in the whole body." He also posited that the retention of sperm could make people lazy and melancholic.

As Foucault notes, there wasn't yet a consensus on the health benefits of abstinence. But the high value placed on sperm during this era popularized the notion that abstaining from sex was a worthwhile exercise, one that athletes practiced to improve their performance and strength.

As you might have guessed, these perks did not extend to women, which is notable given that women now bear most of the pressure to abstain from sex—a major tenet of purity culture that has also, coincidentally, been medicalized. (Evangelical leaders have long suggested that if you have sex before marriage, you could suffer from psychological disorders for the rest of your life, in addition to disappointing the Lord. The reality is, purity culture causes more lasting psychological harm than consensual sexual acts ever could.)[1]

Foucault notes that while sexual abstinence was not yet presumed morally good, nor was sex considered evil, a shift in medical and philosophical thought of the fourth century resulted in "a certain inflection": the insistence on the "peculiar fragility" and "pathogenic power" of sex, and "a valorization of abstinent behaviors, for both sexes."

I dwell on this era not just because it's funny to me that sperm was considered phlegm. Rather, Foucault so convincingly situates the period as the beginning of the *souci de soi,* or the "care of self," that would continue to cloud conversations about sex, both personal and societal—gradually, our sexual choices became linked to goodness and worth.

Fast-forward several hundred years to present day—past Renaissance chastity belts, past witch trials, past Victorian hysteria wards, past the sexual revolution, past the Britney-Madonna-Xtina kiss at the 2003 VMAs. As outlined in chapter 2, the continued supremacy of purity culture and its fixation on extramarital abstinence colors the conversations we have about abstinence today. Many people have internalized the idea that abstaining from sex is morally good, or conversely, that it is problematic due to its religious associations. In case it hasn't already become painfully clear, like can't-take-your-eyes-off-the-car-crash clear, I'm not too concerned with morality, in this book or elsewhere. For this reason alone, or perhaps in conjunction with my mental illnesses, I never internalized shame or guilt about casual sex, despite all the social messaging. And yet, standing proudly in my sexual promiscuity, amid a society determined to punish me for it, I missed out on so many of the benefits of not having sex, the first one being: the freedom that comes from not having sex that wastes your fucking time.

Because to stop having bad sex, or to strive for less of it, you must first understand what role sex plays in your life. This detective work becomes easier when you have some distance from sex, as counterintuitive as that may seem. Consider making a "Why Do I Have Sex?" pie chart. You may notice many of the things you crave from sex are not sex-specific, and can be found in other places that are less likely to waste your time and deplete your energy.

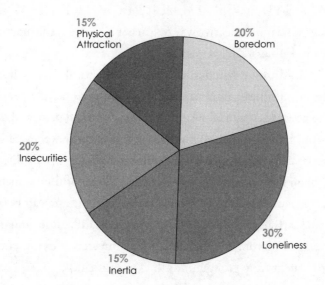

REASONS I HAVE SEX

15% Physical Attraction

20% Boredom

20% Insecurities

30% Loneliness

15% Inertia

While it's futile to try to eliminate all "unnecessary" sex from your life (what is necessary sex, even, besides sex offered by Pedro Pascal), the benefits of intentional dry spells, extended periods of solitude, and solo masturbation are numerous, and more and more young people are embracing conscious bouts of abstinence to reset and recenter, finding that it offers emotional and physical clarity.

Periods of sexual inactivity offer an ideal backdrop to develop a mindfulness practice—perhaps the most crucial solo activity, with benefits that spill over into both your sex life and your ability to understand it. Mindfulness means a lot of things to a lot of people, but in short, it's the ability to perceive the present moment without judgment—just awareness. "To assess the source of your sexual frustration, dissatisfaction, or distress, it's helpful to observe that distress neutrally, without judgment, worry, or upset. Which is a learnable skill," Emily Nagoski advises in her very excellent manual, *The Come As You Are Workbook*. "The most effective way to learn it is through the practice of mindfulness."

"Mindfulness-based interventions," like regular meditation and mindfulness courses, have been shown to benefit people who are suffering from relationship issues, sexual pain, and the lasting impact of sexual trauma.[2] Meditation centers around the country offer group classes for practicing mindfulness, through deep breathing, meditation, and mindful movement. In women, specifically, group mindfulness therapy can boost sexual satisfaction while reducing orgasmic difficulties and depressive symptoms.[3] (People suffering from erectile dysfunction also benefit from group mindfulness treatment.)[4]

You don't have to abstain from sex to practice mindfulness, but solitude enhances this practice. Being alone opens us up for self-discovery and peace in a way that relationships with others cannot. (Again, please disregard this if you are Pedro Pascal; I think we are compatible and just want a chance.) Mindfulness practices hinge on one's relationship with oneself, though the benefits of those practices ultimately enrich our relationship with others, too.

If you're having problems in bed, you need to start outside of the sexual context, says sex and relationship coach Pamela Joy. This starts with just you and your body. Before even touching the topic of partnered sex or even masturbation, Joy encourages clients to practice being mindful of their sensory experiences, and asking questions like: "How do I relate to my body? What possibilities do I allow for? It's about raising awareness around sensory aspects of what it's like to be in a human body."

Tasting, touching, smelling, listening, seeing. While on the phone, she tells me that she's gazing out her bedroom window, noticing the ivy covering the tree, watching the breeze move through branches. She tells me she feels the softness of the velvet blanket beneath her.

"I'm hoping clients notice what it is like when they focus on the awareness of the senses," she said. "Are you sad? Are you happy? Are you excited? Are you angry? What does it do to your body? Does it make you more relaxed? Does it shift something for you?" She explores her clients' relationships with the sensory world long before they start talking about sex. This is solitary work.

Char Adams, the culture writer and friend of mine who has

spent a lifetime unlearning purity culture, committed to this process in a powerful way. She stopped having sex entirely for four years of her twenties, realizing that the sex she was having was unsatisfying and demoralizing. Opting out of sex for an extended stretch can offer a powerful reset, crystallizing perspective that helps you honor your sexual desires, which are too often obscured by other people's desires.

"I was just like, 'Okay, I am going to take time off and really explore this because I do not feel good about having sex that I don't enjoy.' I didn't feel good about not having autonomy and some semblance of power," she told me. "Now is the first time I feel like, 'Oh, I'm having sex because I'm choosing, and I'm enjoying the sex that I'm choosing.' Do you know how empowering that is, that I enjoy choosing to have sex, and that I enjoy it? I chose a partner who wants me to be empowered. Too many women and trans folks are not conditioned to feel empowered and in control."

≋ ≋

I live alone with my Chihuahua, Bucatina, and we are both anxious. The shelter told me she was rescued from a Texas puppy mill, where at the age of three and a half she'd already had at least two litters. She has PTSD and so do I.

Our first few weeks together, I would occasionally host an on-again, off-again hookup for sex and companionship. He and I were both extremely careful recluses (it was early pandemic) who figured that we, too, deserved human contact, just like people who lived with partners.

Bucatina does not bark. When she is scared—from triggers such as clapping, fireworks, and skateboarding youths—she trembles so fiercely that she forgets to breathe. The last time this friend came to my apartment for sex, and the last time I had sex before kicking off the longest dry spell of my adult life, was the first time I had sex with Bucatina in the apartment. It was already distressing enough to her that a strange man sat next to me on the couch seat she had clearly claimed by repeatedly vomiting on the cushion. But when the man and I migrated to the bed, she tried to hop in, perching her little head on the corner of the mattress and pushing her snout into the mix as best she could. When the man lowered himself on top of me, Bucatina barked hysterically. How is a dog to know what human sex looks like, and that it is not murder? Without the proper conceptual framework, the scene looked violent; I get it. We continued having sex, assuming she would eventually calm down, but she didn't. I hopped on top and that seemed to placate her, though the trembling continued. I could now count at least five things preoccupying my brain while getting dicked: 1) Traumatizing Bucatina. 2) My neck acne, now on full display due to the position. 3) My shoddily built bed frame, which would indeed collapse moments later. 4) That time twenty years ago at summer camp when I tried out referring to my period as "my PD" to make it seem cool that I'd had it. 5) Hunger for SunChips.

I was not mindful of the sensations in my body. Rather, my mind was yanked in a million directions. Even in the years before I had a Chihuahua fully unraveling beside me during sex acts, my mind had no trouble yanking itself to other matters—perhaps to SunChips, or to my eventual death.

I should have taken Bucatina's advice. The man wasn't attacking me, nor was I in danger of physical harm, but I was having sex for reasons that warranted pause, and was far too preoccupied to enjoy it. This was someone I'd been attempting to stop sleeping with for over a year. A year! The emotional whiplash of our relationship—being friends who had sex when we were bored—did not feel "healthy" or "good," even though I wanted to feel like I could tolerate breezy sex arrangements like the punk rocker I fancy myself to be. It also became clear to me that I wouldn't be able to enjoy sex, or sink into the moment enough to orgasm, if I didn't figure out how to get out of my head and back into my body. On a technical level, there was nothing *wrong* with the sex we were having. But it was bad sex, because I was miserable.

That was the last time I had sex for almost a year. The more time that passed, the more it felt like it could be the last time ever, which I knew was Bucatina's deepest held wish. It has felt remarkable to be writing a book about sex when, for most of the process, I struggled to recall what sex was. But even more remarkable is the way this dry spell helped rehabilitate my relationship with sex. Not only am I now more likely to gravitate toward masturbation when horniness strikes, rather than text someone who chronically disappoints me—giving me the benefits of sex without the pesky agonizing—but I have restructured my standard for having partnered sex, in a way that feels validating and compassionate to both myself and my Chihuahua.

This isn't to say I'm not starved for touch, or that I don't fantasize about sex with every tall person I pass in the streets, but I feel far more equipped with the tools, vocabulary, and sense of self that are prereqs for pleasurable sexual experiences.

Ideally, long periods of sexual reflection are not spurred by a global pandemic, but the circumstances have allowed me to stop and consider my hopes for a sexual partner—something I'd never done before. Can you do these reflections when you're not in a dry spell? Yes. But I've found, as have many sex therapists, that when you take away the pressure of sexual activity, it's easier to go inward. Here's a recent checklist of my sexual hopes and dreams, something I'd never have taken the time to do were I not languishing in isolation.

1. I want to feel emotionally safe with my sexual partners.
2. I would like for my sexual partners not to draw from high school debate experience to argue against condoms.
3. I will speak up if my leg falls asleep.
4. I will stop 69'ing as a treat for others.
5. I will not have sex with anyone who brings up the goings on of podcast hosts.
6. I will lock Bucatina in the bathroom with her toys during future sexual encounters.
7. I will not tolerate fingering without clitoral stimulation.
8. I will build a bed frame that does not crash to the floor every fifth night.
9. I will incorporate vibrators into sex.
10. I will try to make peace with the body parts I hate, starting most urgently with the area where my thighs meet my knees.

Make your list. When was the last time you took a beat to determine what you wanted out of sex and romance? Maybe the last time was playing MASH at summer camp and writing your crush under the future husband category "as a joke" while praying you ended up with him and not Mr. Peanut.

In our ever-optimized, efficiency-obsessed society, we bring a calculating intentionality to most domains of our life: work, exercise, reading goals. For all the worrying we do about sex, and sex-adjacent matters like pubic hair presentation, we often don't bring this consciousness to our own desire, which deepens with mindfulness and independent reflection. Understanding our sex lives, unfortunately, requires personal excavating. Too often the very real needs and wants that drive us to sex—attachment issues, self-esteem issues, ennui, rage—obscure the act so profoundly that we accept, expect, and even seek out mediocre sex, in turn dragging us even further from sexual happiness. If we stopped demanding so much of sex, or at least understood our demands (maybe to pass the time, or feel alive) might we feel more empowered to appreciate and pursue the full spectrum of activities that bring us closer to what we actually want and enjoy, which is often not sex?

Many people I've spoken with have found themselves stuck within dry spells they did not choose and actively resent. More uncomfortable than the lack of sex, to them, is the anxiety surrounding this absence—the sense that they should be having more, that more means healthy, that the perceived scarcity of sex reflected poorly on their relationships. One man told me in an informal survey about their sex life, "I want to want to have more! But that's probably just society telling me I should have more, idk." Idk either, guy. It's hard to k.

Not to be a cool pastor sitting backward on a chair to hype Jesus, but the sick thing about dry spells, whether they're intentional or not, is they can help you recalibrate your relationship with sex, in the same way that giving up alcohol for a month offers insights into your relationship with drinking that you couldn't have accessed otherwise.

Extreme solitude begets reflection. For many single people, especially those who live alone, sex vanished from the menu during the pandemic, because it became exponentially more difficult to coordinate. For many partnered people, sex vanished, too; the pandemic has soured people's libidos. So now that we're here, what can we learn?

Carol Queen is a sexologist and founding director of the legendary San Francisco sex shop Good Vibrations. On a dreary January evening, quite close to the anniversary of my last penetration, we spoke on the phone. A prolific author of erotica and books on sexual wellness since the 1970s, Queen is credited with helping popularize the idea of "sex-positivity."

Queen and I chatted about consent, communication, and the lessons of kink. Like most conversations during the pandemic, the existential stakes felt high. I wanted to know: What will After look like? Will we be okay? What is anything? Trying to be a little more pleasant, I told her that not having sex for such a long time had helped me realize certain truths about myself. I paused. Did she think this was true? Did she think I was growing? Did she think I would be okay? WOULD I BE OKAY?

Queen felt: yes. She suggested that the distance from sex, that many people have been thrust into during the pandemic, could foster growth, especially if you leaned into it.

"If somebody is introspective, this is bound to be a reset moment," she told me. "Whether that means that they back away from sex, whether that means that they get clearer about what might have been problematic in the first place, whether it's a matter of retuning expectations. This situation is allowing us to ask ourselves some questions."

The answer to most of these questions—and she has been asked thousands over her career—is "know thyself." It's an answer that, unfortunately, requires more questions.

"Know what you want, know what you've gone to—you know, the people you find the most attractive or compatible—and let yourself understand and accept the way you're wired right now. Know that it might get more fluid later. It might change to something else," she said. "Maybe on the other side, it will be easier for people to talk about the way that they confronted ideas that they had about what sex was supposed to be, what relationships were supposed to look like. Maybe they started to find their own personal dream of it, because it's not going to be the same for everybody."

This internal interrogation happens on two levels: there's the macro-mindfulness of thinking about your sex life more holistically: what you're looking for, what you've hated, what you want to try before you die. And then there's the more granular mindfulness: cultivating an awareness of the present moment where you accept all passing feelings, thoughts, and sensations without overidentifying with them.

For the former, problem-solving requires awareness of the problem. One tool is communicating with people you trust to listen without judgment, like close friends, loved ones, therapists, and dogs. But the best and easiest place to start is with a gel pen and a notebook. (It doesn't have to be a gel pen, but I've found I'm more inclined to journal when the ink is silky smooth.)

Queen is adamantly pro-journaling, both about sex and the universe.

"Journaling is great because you're basically talking to yourself, letting yourself know what you already know inside, and maybe won't get real about quite yet," she said. "It's that process of bringing stuff to the surface. To me, it's either the next best thing or the best thing compared to seeing a therapist."

Let's say you're in a dry spell. Maybe it's intentional, maybe it's not, but you now have lots of extra time on your hands and maybe some anxiety about not having sex. Maybe you've gotten it into your head that everyone else is having so much sex and just, like, loving it. You order a notebook and a gel pen and tell yourself you'll start journaling when the items arrive but not a moment before. It arrives quickly and you're like, fuck, do I have to journal now? You spend the day drawing hearts and those cartoon block *s*'s from middle school. Weeks go by. The seasons change. A new hair sprouts on your jawline. Okay, okay. Finally, you decide, you're ready to start journaling. You sit down. You get up to grab coffee. Another week passes. You sit down again and are ready to start for real. Where do you begin?

"If you're journaling, you get the opportunity to write out adventures you've had where you wonder why you thought you were going to have a certain kind of experience and it wound up that you had a really different one," said Queen. "When I was a young slut, somebody would be very polite and ask, 'What do you like?' And I'd be like, 'Oh, anything.' What was I doing? I was trying to learn more about what sex was, because I didn't actually know much yet. I was on the right track. Although I was also lucky because it could have been more dicey than it was. And sometimes it's dicey, right?"

Recently, for the first time ever, I wrote down the name of every person I've slept with (or a few descriptor words, like "chode private equity"). I've always resisted the exercise because tallying sexual partners feels like a "kill count"–type deal, putting an importance on the number of partners—a metric we're taught is significant from a young age but that is fundamentally meaningless. (One of my all-time favorite studies, by which I mean one that wakes me in the night to dry-sob, found that both men and women are more attracted to people who've had fewer sexual partners.)[5]

I found the list-making oddly comforting, if at times unsettling. (Yes, things can be both: for example, six Pop-Tarts for dinner.) As is true of most journaling, expelling the contents of your brain onto a page facilitates a healthy release. You can assess words on a page far easier than thoughts in a skull, and the process becomes less agonizing, too—in the same way to-do lists are less overwhelming when they're written down, rather than floating untethered in your consciousness. There was no plan to be made of my sex list—more of a to-did list than a to-do list—but it triggered feelings of compassion I can't always access in my dealings with free-floating memories. Past Maria didn't have anything better to do at 11:05 P.M. on a Tuesday night than sleep with "chode private equity." I will hold her in the light.

👁 👁

One thirty-year-old cis straight woman told me she'd been celibate for three of the past four years. (She lost her "second virginity," as she and her friends called it, this year.) After a painful breakup, she slipped into an unintentional abstinence—she lacked the confidence to put herself out there and pursue anything romantic. But after the first year, she found that she "didn't miss partnered sex much," she told me. "I was living for slow-burning flirtations with people who lived in other cities, or with people with whom I had hot and cold flirtations . . . I did find my 'dry spell' was turning into something more intentional, comfortable, and safe—especially since I was continuing to have satisfying sex on my own."

When she finally did decide to sleep with someone, the experience was satisfying and fun. "I am someone who would rather just not have sex with other people unless I'm really into them, because I feel comfortable and satisfied just having sex with myself for long periods of time," she told me. "Hell, I made it those three years, what's another few months when there's no one satisfying in the picture?"

For people in relationships, dry spelling becomes more complicated. There tends to be an expectation that you have sex with your romantic partner, though this is not always true: asexual romantic relationships are intimate and complete without sex, as are other relationships where sex is understood to be off the table, for whatever reason. Nonetheless, there's still an enormous amount of pressure placed on sex within relationships, with frequency presumed to be a barometer of healthiness. If you're having no sex, or less sex than what you imagine is normal, you worry the relationship is broken. The tension intensifies when libidos are mismatched within monogamous relationships—one person feels deprived and unwanted; the other feels pressured, guilty, or even coerced. This imbalance is called a "desire discrepancy," or "desire mismatch," and it's quite common.[6] The more time that passes without an honest conversation about the mismatch, the more the fault lines calcify into resentments, like the ones you'll find on the Reddit page r/deadbedrooms, where people with high libidos commiserate about their low-libido partners. One post is entitled "Resentful that she makes me come to bed early with no hope of sex."

Within a monogamous relationship, the idea that each person's sex drive should sync up perfectly is far-fetched, yet commonly expected: *We have sex this number of times per week because we both want to have sex that number of times per week and we feel good about everything. No one is ever repulsed by anyone, especially not anyone who gets yogurt all over their lips every time they eat yogurt, which is often. Everyone is fine with that. We're fine! We have sex.*

Sometimes couples who aren't having sex do, in fact, hate

each other and should break up. But attraction is complicated, fickle. Taking sex off the table is one way to not only encourage individual exploration and mindfulness, but to engineer some spark.

One classic formula for sexual interest is attraction + obstacles = excitement. So what if the attraction is there, but there are no obstacles? As in: you think your boyfriend is mostly attractive (barring quarantine novelty mustache), but you live together and are painfully aware that he is always DTF. So, no excitement. Or maybe, the obstacles are there, but the attraction isn't! As in: he lives far away, but you think he's ugly. So, no excitement.

It's tricky to manufacture attraction. Presumably some base amount is there if you got into the relationship, but people's feelings change. If excitement is the problem, throwing obstacles into the mix can get things moving. One sexual obstacle is choosing not to have sex for a predetermined length of time. This is a classic sex therapy exercise for a reason: if you're surrounded by your partner, if there is no distance, there is no excitement. Cut to resentment cycle, cut to bad sex—having sex you don't want just to placate your partner and buy more time. Spending sexual time alone alleviates some of the pressure we put on partnered sex.

"Working on your sexuality really starts as an inside job," Pamela Joy told me. She sometimes suggests her partnered clients take sex off the table for a month and observe what comes up. "For someone to start their exploration of sexuality, they have to focus on learning more about themselves before they focus on what's happening between them and an existing partner."

It's useful to think about intimacy beyond sex. Julian Gavino, a trans model and activist with Ehlers-Danlos syndrome, speaks openly about sex and disability on his Instagram page, which has over sixty-nine thousand followers. Gavino, who is a sexual assault survivor, hasn't always had a breezy relationship with sex, but for the most part, he's found sex to be pleasurable, even throughout a fraught ten-year relationship, during which he came out as trans and learned, at eighteen, that he would be wheelchair-bound for the rest of his life. Disability fundamentally transformed his relationship to sex, forcing him to explore other ways to feel intimate both during sex and at times he didn't feel up to having it. On days Gavino doesn't have the energy for sex, but still wants to feel connected to his partner, he taps into a well of other intimate activities. Within relationships, the pressure to have sex can override the desire to say no. The result? Unpleasant sex.

"It's about finding alternate ways to still be intimate. Maybe one day I don't have the capacity to do a whole thing," he said, "so maybe we'll just mutually masturbate together. Or some sort of cuddling or massage." Another activity he's enjoyed, that he fully recognizes is not for everyone, is staring into his partner's eyes for several minutes, both unclothed. Just as important as feeling comfortable with sex as we'd ordinarily define it—interacting with someone else's body, and vice versa, in a way that feels intimate—is realizing there's a universe beyond sex that can be equally gratifying and intimate.

Many people in relationships describe the sex they don't particularly want to have—but offer for the sake of their partner—as a sort of maintenance work, meant to boost morale. Sex as maintenance is a pretty mundane reality for countless couples whose sex drives don't sync up perfectly. Emily Nagoski, the sex educator and author of *Come as You Are,* classifies sex as an "attachment behavior," so it makes sense we have it to reinforce our relationships. But it's not the only behavior that can soothe attachment insecurity or foster connection. Too often we're unwilling to explore the full spectrum of non-sex activities that also fulfill our desire for intimacy.

Even when we're not in the mood, we have sex with people we care about or like some amount, if we feel the attachment is threatened. Over time, this routine of appeasing via sex can erode the foundation of our sexual selves, and it can carry over into the actual sex. In *The Pleasure Gap,* Katherine Rowland likens the impulse to prioritize a partner's sexual desire over one's own—for example, by faking an orgasm or having sex at all—as an act of caretaking, a dynamic many women are pressured to perform from a young age. There's a hitch, though, and a big one: many women Rowland interviewed "assumed responsibility for managing the emotional outcome of the sexual interaction, even if that meant temporarily subordinating their disappointments, pain, or disinterest." She continued, "As we act out ecstasy, we devalue our actual sensations. On the one hand, this performance is an ode to the importance of female pleasure, the expectation that it should be present. But on the other, it strips women of the physical and psychological experience of pleasure. Spectacle bullies sensation aside." [7]

To opt out of sex we don't feel like having, and to avoid the trap of performing during it, we must build a vocabulary for communicating our wants and needs, even when they don't sync up with a partner's.

"I realized that for me, being trans and disabled, I'm going to need to be able to really communicate directly with someone before, during, and after sex," Gavino told me. "I learned to find my voice and speak up by saying, yes, I do need to schedule sex. Or if I have to stop having sex for pain, or if I don't like something, I'm going to speak up. It continues to be a process." There are other ways to maintain intimacy besides sex. They just require practice.

Masturbation, which we'll ~touch~ next, is a crucial tool for deepening sexual satisfaction and awareness, with partners and oneself. It's easy to fall into the trap of understanding your sexuality only through the lens of partnered sex. Your body is yours to enjoy, first and foremost. The sexual relationship you have with yourself matters more than the one you have with anyone else.

5

THE TRANSFORMATIVE POWER
OF MASTURBATION

"Don't wait for me; I can't come."

—*Mitski*

Despite its horrors, I love *The Bachelor*. It's one of my simplest pleasures, like telling my dog she's a baby. I don't, however, find it romantic or aspirational. I don't swoon watching them soar above western Pennsylvania in hot-air balloons, or make out in front of fireworks while their perfectly staged chicken marsalas go cold. Rather, the thrill for me is watching such a succinct, albeit unhinged, portrait of contemporary culture and all the micro-performances, on camera and off, that make up a life. Given the premise of the show—thirty people will do whatever it takes to marry a stranger—the insights on sex and romance are particularly revealing: on display are all the norms we inhale and metabolize whether we want to or not, whether we know better or not, because we live in a society.

On the first episode of every *Bachelor* or *Bachelorette*, contestants looking for love and toothbrush sponsorships arrive at the mansion in limos. They briefly introduce themselves to the romantic lead before heading inside to the "cocktail party," the first of many nights wherein the producers systematically deprive contestants of sleep to engineer drama. Occasionally, a contestant pierces through the noise, and on Matt James's scandal-ridden season, it was Katie Thurston, a woman who showed up with a vibrator as her conversation piece (and later went on to become the bachelorette).

Unlike the emotional abuse exacted by producers, or the graphic boob grazing in hot tubs, the vibrator was censored. You may not have even identified it as a vibrator were it not blurred, which signifies inappropriateness; sexuality often becomes recognizable by its coding as improper. Mentally, the viewer had to reverse engineer the vibrator, starting with the blur and going backward. Throughout the show, fellow castmates repeatedly referred to the vibrator as a "dildo"—a revealing imprecision of language not unlike calling a vulva a vagina.* The girls in the house expressed discomfort, even disgust, with the vibrator, just like the producers who blurred it, in accordance with network guidelines. In one scene, a contestant complains to a group of girls about Katie, saying, "The way that she came in hella-hot with her sex-positivity . . . ," putting sex-positivity in air quotes, her tone disdainful, as though being sex-positive was the grossest thing you could be (besides here for the wrong reasons).

*In recent years, there has been a movement among sex educators to refer to the vulva not as a "vagina," as it is commonly called, but as what it is: a vulva. The word "vagina" signifies only the reproductive canal, not the entire genital apparatus. Imagine calling your nose a nasal cavity, or your ear a Eustachian tube. Why should we reduce intricate genitalia to just one tiny part that is famously relevant to penis insertion?

To be abundantly clear, a vibrator's sole purpose is to provide pleasure to genitals. What about that is disgusting? And why does the mere existence of a vibrator exceed the threshold of appropriateness?

Masturbation is taboo, arguably more taboo than sex itself, and the stigma of self-pleasure reliably interferes with our sexual well-being. While masturbation could not be more natural (as pleasure-drunk babies, we touch ourselves constantly), learning that other people masturbate, and that it's normal, good, and healthy, is a process that takes far longer than it needs to, wreaking havoc in its wake. Over the course of our sexual and emotional development, we are left to figure out masturbation on our own, with some help from unrealistic porn, but not before internalizing that we are sick freaks for doing it, or that it's a depressing substitute for REAL sex.

Masturbation is a vital pathway to transforming our sexual relationships with others, ourselves, and the universe. Because to understand and transform our sex lives, we must first understand and transform our relationship with self-pleasure—good sex starts with us.

Ash, a twenty-eight-year-old queer, trans sex educator, is a vehement masturbation enthusiast. It's no coincidence, then, that they are one of the few people I spoke with while researching this book who is deeply satisfied with their sex life. The satisfaction extends far beyond the scope of sex; self-connection is transformative. Masturbation gave Ash a blueprint to map sexual encounters into deeply pleasurable ones.

"Masturbation was the first sex I ever had, and it's responsible for probably eighty percent of my lifetime orgasms," they told me. "Because of touching myself, I know how I like to be touched, and can teach other people. I know what I like to think about when I get myself off, which has informed the fantasies I share and act out with other people. But as I've gotten older and the quality and intimacy of my partnered sex has improved, my masturbation has morphed from a necessary sexual outlet to an—even more necessary—outlet for stress relief that has very little to do with my sex life."

When they are feeling sexual, they have sex with their partner. But when they're feeling "stressed, or dissociated, or disconnected from my body, or grumpy, or when I'm dealing with chronic illness pain or period pain," they masturbate. "Either way," Ash said, "it's an invaluable self-connection that I don't plan to ever give up."

For many of us whose partnered sex remains largely unsatisfying, focusing our attention on solo sex knocks two big action items off our list: we can both learn to enjoy being in our bodies more (making it easier to opt out of bad partnered sex) *and* improve the partnered sex we are having, as we'll know what to ask for.

In fact, masturbation is such a powerful tool that many sex therapists hinge their work on it entirely. Amy Weissfeld, a certified sex educator, works as a masturbation coach, helping her clients reform their relationship to self-pleasure and see beyond the frenzied drive to orgasm. Part of her work, she says, is broadening the definition of masturbation to include self-pleasure of all kinds, even acts like the stroke of a cheek. She urges her clients to move away from an outcome-obsessed model that centers on orgasm, which gets us in our heads and out of our bodies.

The matter is personal for Weissfeld, who had a sexual re-awakening in her late thirties. "I needed to reclaim myself before I could bring myself into my relationship with my partner in a wholesome, full way," she told me. "When we expand the definition of what masturbation is, it allows us to really feel embodied and to love ourselves. And when we start to love ourselves, we're so much more powerful and radiant."

Weissfeld believes that masturbation will "heal the world," one person at a time.

꙳ ꙳

You probably learned to be embarrassed by sex toys and masturbation long before you started watching *The Bachelor,* and if you never started watching *The Bachelor,* congratulations, you're a fucking intellectual, but you learned somewhere else. When we are young, we are horny detectives patching together clues, little snippets from conversations or Snapchats or movies, to fill in the gaps of information we aren't getting at school or anywhere else: a blurred vibrator on primetime; a serial killer on a crime procedural who ejaculates on his victims; a young Jason Biggs pleasuring himself with a pie to experience mortification so massive it titles a feature film. Many kids are scolded when they first start touching themselves. Yes, I forgive your mom for yelling "GO TO YOUR ROOM" when she caught seven-year-old you humping the one nice couch pillow; masturbation is private, unless shared with consenting parties. But the act of rubbing, pulling, stroking, and tapping your genitals could not be more natural. Alas, there comes a time in every masturbator's life, usually during childhood, when we internalize that it is wrong. It could be when your mom yelled at you, which cemented a lifelong association between self-pleasure and humiliation. Or it could be a literal educator saying, "Masturbation can cause blindness," which is still taught in some classrooms, I learned.

Most people I spoke with figured out how to masturbate on their own, but couldn't pinpoint when. Years after this initial discovery, these same masturbators told me they still never talk about it with friends, family, or even (especially!) significant others. In relationships, there's a pervasive fear that if you're masturbating too often or even at all, your partner might conclude that sex with them is not enough, or even consider it cheating.

The messages we glean from pop culture, peers, church, and our families—that masturbation is humiliating, gross—hold extra weight because we aren't learning about our bodies elsewhere. One of the biggest shortcomings of American sex education, with its laser-focus on the absolute worst things that could happen to you, is its failure to acknowledge that genital stimulation is pleasurable. That sex is pleasurable, that touching your genitals feels good. While boys at least get the message that they are insatiable little sex hounds, at formative ages, girls and gender-expansive adolescents don't learn that sex should feel good, cementing a standard for years (or a lifetime) of sexual experiences that don't feel good. Many adults experience guilt before, during, and after masturbation well into adulthood.[1]

With few other resources, our sex education is porn, where masturbation is usually an erotic performance for others.

Gen Z and millennials are the first generations whose sexual educations are largely internet-driven. While past generations faced similar or worse educational shortcomings, young people today have new opportunities to fill those gaps with online miscellany—but often without the critical media literacy skills to navigate messaging, or to parse out: *In porn, when women masturbate, they scream in a sexy, breathy way, and they squirt everywhere. It's normal and okay, however, that when I masturbate, I not only don't squirt, but need lube for moisture, and I not only don't scream in a sexy, breathy way, but squeal like a raccoon stuck in a trash can.*

If porn is your first and only consistent exposure to other people's labias, how will you come to feel about your own large, not smooth, and uneven labia? Will you feel comfortable when you play with it? Will you turn off the negative self-chatter long enough to find sexual satisfaction, alone or with a partner?

Big Mouth, an animated Netflix series, chronicles the indignities of pubescence. In an episode about masturbation, Andrew Glouberman, a hyper-horny middle schooler voiced by John Mulaney, demonstrates to his friend what he calls "the Glouberman method" for jerking off—"a delicate dance in just seventeen steps." The obsessive ritual involves locking his bedroom door, dimming the lights, putting on music, lowering the shades, flipping over bedside photos of his parents and the Mets, readying a Lululemon maternity catalogue, double-checking the lock, pulling out tissues, pumping three squirts of lotion, taking off his pants, triple-checking the lock. When his friend interrupts him, Glouberman has to start over from the beginning. Everything must be just so.

What *Big Mouth* does so well is shine a humorous light on the unspoken so it doesn't feel so dark anymore, letting us know: *Hey, everyone is hugely embarrassing. No one is alone in this*. I could have used that growing up. Like most of the country's sexual education, my curriculum did not cover pleasure, self-generated or otherwise. Sex was a dangerous yet inevitable *situation* that would befall me because of incorrigible boys. The closest we got to "pleasure" was wet dreams, a thing that happened to boys in the night that I only learned years later was categorically different from peeing.

I spoke with one thirty-seven-year-old cis-het mother of three who didn't begin masturbating until her mid-twenties, after her husband encouraged her to try it. She still doesn't understand what had blocked her from ever exploring masturbation on her own. "Probably buried Catholic guilt—that I didn't even know or acknowledge," she said. (Numerous religions consider masturbation a sin, including Roman Catholicism, Eastern Orthodox, Oriental Orthodox, and many strains of Protestantism.) She's still somewhat confused by her reticence to masturbate, given that her parents were so open and liberal. "Especially my mom. She would never dream of shaming any of us for that. But it's so deeply rooted in the culture."

A 2011 study found that young adults' feelings toward masturbation were shaped by the social stigma and taboo surrounding self-pleasure—nearly all the study's participants learned about masturbation through the media and their peers, rather than at school or at home. The study acknowledges masturbation "as a strategy to improve sexual health, promote relational intimacy, and reduce unwanted pregnancy, STIs, and HIV transmission" and a key part of healthy sexual development. While men still internalized the stigma of masturbation to some degree, they were far more likely to recognize the benefits of doing it than women, who struggled to accept it as normal or acceptable.[2]

Then, it makes sense that, as adults, we remain cagey about masturbation. While the shame surrounding it may be gendered—in a way that disproportionately discourages people with vulvas—many men I spoke with had complicated feelings, too, though they reported masturbating regularly. A thirty-year-old cis-het man, who I'll call Ryan, told me he masturbates almost every day, but doesn't particularly enjoy it. It feels like a chore.

"I've been told that masturbation helps your sex life, but personally I haven't found that," he said. "It seems stale and a waste of time. I mean, I've been masturbating the same way since I was, like, thirteen. What else in my life have I been doing the same way and still find it effective?"

Another thirty-year-old cis-het man, who I'll call Bryan because he's just like Ryan, echoed this sentiment. He masturbates three or four times a week but wishes it were less. He has no positive feelings about masturbating. He wishes he didn't have to "rely on self-service" that required "smutty videos."

"Sex is a lot better than masturbation and involves actual intimacy instead," he said. "Masturbation has a role for me in an ideally sexually diversified lifestyle, but it's a small part." I asked him if he thought sex with others was more intimate than sex with himself. "I've never really considered intimacy something that can happen by oneself. There's no interpersonal joy that comes from being with myself. I still enjoy it, but I don't feel closer to myself for having wanked it, you know?"

Regardless of how you internalized the message that masturbating is lesser than partnered sex, or even the idea, like Ryan, that it is a tedious exercise, this reluctance blocks us from pleasure.

Masturbating is one of the healthiest things we can do for ourselves and our sex lives. And it's free! Most of the materials we need come complimentary with birth. Self-pleasuring releases feel-good hormones like dopamine and oxytocin, and can help us rehabilitate our understandably fraught relationship with pleasure, reduce stress, and build affirming sexual fantasies.[3] Our reluctance to explore self-pleasure robs us of a valuable tool for developing sexual autonomy. Ryan is masturbating, but he doesn't care for himself the way he cares for sexual partners.

Amy Weissfeld, the sex coach, recalls masturbating as a child—"babies are pleasure seekers," she told me repeatedly—but then dropping it for years. Nothing dramatic happened, but she became busy with other things, and self-pleasure plummeted to the bottom of the to-do list.

"I was in a good relationship and I just got busy doing other things. Like, life happened, and it didn't seem important," she said. "My partner would say to me, 'What do you want? What do you like?' And I'd be like, 'I don't know, whatever you're doing is fine. It's all good.' I was dissociated from my body because of all this body shame."

It wasn't until she expanded her own definition of masturbation into a broader practice of self-pleasure, one that wasn't so orgasm-obsessed, that she stepped into her sexuality. She began touching herself like she was someone she loved.

"What was key to my own sexuality was recognizing, number one, the importance of masturbation, but number two, that masturbation doesn't have to be rubbing on the clit till I have an orgasm," she said. "What I try to get people to do is not focus on trying to ejaculate or trying to have an orgasm or trying to perform in some way, but to just experience pleasure in the body. So sometimes, for me, I might just sit there with my hand on my heart for thirty minutes and I meditate. It's like an erotic meditation. I'm redefining masturbation as self-love."

〰 〰

I spent a recent afternoon jerking off a woman with my computer cursor. My hands clammy with sweat, I rubbed the white arrow up, across, and down her clitoris, just as she had instructed me in a tutorial video. "Accent one part, just like that," Diana said breathily. Her vulva spread across my whole screen; I could see the contours of every shaved hair follicle. When I moved my cursor across the clit, the skin rippled to reflect the pressure. The level of realism almost disturbed me: I was interacting with an item that I have owned, on my body, for over three decades, yet have never properly investigated.

On the recommendation of a sex therapist I interviewed, I was perusing OMGYes.com, an encyclopedia of masturbation techniques and tips for people with vulvas, featuring instructional (and graphic) videos, animations, and diagrams of moves to enhance pleasure. The original series highlights twelve "ingredients to enhance pleasure," drawing from the collective wisdom of two thousand cis women aged eighteen to ninety-five. There are twelve modules you can explore, each with videos of women talking about a specific technique, ranging from edging to "orbiting" (which is exactly what it sounds like—the clitoris is the sun, your finger a planet), and demonstrating on their own vulvas.

I started with the "accenting" module. "Accenting" is their term for upgrading a repetitive motion by adding extra pressure to one portion of the movement. You can "accent" a down stroke, an up stroke, or a segment of a circle. "Pleasure isn't symmetrical—and giving the clit more or less attention on different areas can actually feel much better than treating all parts the same," the video description reads. I felt attacked! I certainly do not grant my clit that degree of nuance. I rub it until what needs to happen happens. When I think about going down on a partner with a penis, or using my hands on someone else—*then,* I have technique! The thoughtfulness with which I handle other people's genitalia, compared to the carelessness with which I handle my own, reminded me of Ryan, the masturbator who speeds through masturbation but takes his sweet time to pleasure others.

I've never been a big masturbator, and it's been a lifelong insecurity. I didn't masturbate as an adolescent, just sort of recreationally touched my vulva around the house, and bystanders were kind enough not to say anything. I only started in college, begrudgingly, because a suitemate found out I didn't and said I had to try it, as though masturbation were Zumba (big at the time). I'd never even seen porn before, so she showed that to me, too. I wasn't moved by the visuals—I couldn't find anything that aroused me the way my own sick thoughts of Alan Rickman did—but I eventually figured out how to touch myself until it felt good.

That good feeling, though, rarely seemed to merit the extreme lengths I had to go to; I require total silence, a peaceful headspace, and nothing on my to-do list for the next several days. Just like Andrew Glouberman, I'm a masturbation diva, crippled by anxiety. I travel with a friend who never leaves the house without her tiny bullet vibrator, and on vacations, we give each other lots of alone time to preserve the friendship. When she leaves the hotel room to grab coffee, I'm lucky if I can successfully use that solo time to take a shit. When I leave the hotel room for coffee, she can get off in less than three minutes. Unlike Ryan, and my masturbation champion of a friend, my issue has never been rushing through it. Most of the time, my anxiety makes any "it" feel impossible. The negative self-chatter dulls all sensation: *When am I going to orgasm? Is this ingrown hair a tumor? When is dinner?*

I hoped that OMGYes would offer some physical stimulation techniques that could help lessen, or at least distract from, that anxiety. To illuminate accenting, an animation demonstrated the technique as applied to the upper left side of the clit. On a zoomed-in sketch of the clitoral hood, a turquoise light traveled up the left side; then the light swelled in size and traveled down that same side, faster. Another animation showed repeating side-to-side motions that pushed harder on the clit when it reached the left side.

In the tutorial video, the woman I would go on to masturbate explained, "It's the hood I'm moving over the clit and not the actual clit itself." She demonstrated drawing a clockwise D around her clit, pressing on the hood. "As it gets closer to the finish line, that's when the [D-shaped motions] get smaller.

That's when I move faster." It becomes a "really intense waltz," she said, until she orgasms.

I spent hours watching technique videos, never in my life having witnessed a vulva experiencing pleasure, undramatized—that is, without the express purpose of arousing a viewer. The exercise was educational, the sort of thing adolescents should do in classrooms, before they turn into thirty-year-olds who must go through the trouble of writing a book to figure out the workings of their genitals.

∽ ∽

As sex experts insist, masturbation is a platform for healing. When sex fails us, as it is wont to do, self-pleasure offers refuge, joy, and, most important, information about our sexual identities. OMGYes.com is just one of many relatively recent initiatives aimed at helping people enhance their regular masturbation practices, offering practical, educational tools.

We don't ordinarily think of pleasure as a practice, but it is, and one with neurological implications: the more we strengthen our pleasure pathways, the easier it becomes for us to access them. (Neuroplasticity, or the brain's ability to rewire itself, goes both ways; it not only wires our body's response to trauma, but can also tweak neural networks to promote well-being, as it does with regular meditation.)[4]

"Mindful masturbation" is a trend that's gaining steam as an antidote to the masturbation anxiety that plagues so many of us. If some tiny part of you still believes masturbation is embarrassing, or if it's something you never felt comfortable enough to do, how can you fully relax into pleasure? If you struggle to experience pleasure alone, when the stakes are low, you're likely struggling to feel pleasure with partners, when you might become preoccupied with performing or looking hot. The idea behind masturbating mindfully is to access the enormous range of pleasurable sensations our bodies are designed to feel, beyond just orgasm.

Sex therapist Pamela Joy encourages clients to explore their relationships with masturbation—often to troubleshoot issues with partnered sex, but more importantly to increase awareness of one's own experience of pleasure. Joy, who says she acts as a "shame detector" during sessions, tells her patients to stay curious about any shame that comes up during masturbation.

After chatting with Joy, I tried mindful masturbation for myself, paying closer attention to my environment: the feeling of my unwashed bedsheets, the quality of the air, the sound of my white noise machine (blasting "summer night"), the smell of lavender oil rubbed on my wrists. I had set my room up like a spa, to the best of my abilities, lighting my favorite candles and cleaning away as much garbage as I could.

I slipped into my favorite robe, a plush, pink one. I lay in bed with a powerful wand vibrator, knowing I had just a few minutes before my Chihuahua would get wise to the fact that I had left our spot on the couch. I didn't have any lube on hand, which is hugely beneficial to masturbation of any kind, but I did have some expired face oil. Could that work? I grabbed my phone out from under my butt and googled "marula oil lube work?" Inconclusive results. Trying to stay flexible and resist derailment, I took a few deep breaths. I checked Instagram quickly and then put my phone on the floor. I tried to center myself in the moment and in my body, laboring to notice the softness of my robe. That morning I'd shaved my entire body, having convinced myself that if I were slick as a dolphin, masturbating would feel more luxurious, and wasn't that the point? To feel like a sleek, fancy little dolphin? Joy suggested stroking my body, my thighs, my breasts, my stomach. I had never touched myself like this before, like a person I loved. Right on cue, panic congregated in my chest. I hoisted myself out of bed to check my front door; it was locked. I live alone, but you never know when a burglar will waltz in and humiliate you. I checked my phone again. I put it away again.

I got back in bed with the wand. Its grumbling vibration was powerful, almost intimidating. I tapped it onto my clit and tried to enjoy myself as Bucatina ran laps around the bed, fearing the worst. I closed my eyes so I could feel, or "see feelingly" as my favorite Peloton yoga instructor likes to say; I started thinking about her, the kind of perfect sex she might have. STOP. I was getting derailed again. Back to square one. I took a few deep breaths. I started again. The sensation of the toy echoing across my vulva was intense and my clit responded quite quickly, sending warmth and tingles through my pelvis. My arms felt warm. I tightened my legs, squeezed my butt, and curled my toes as it buzzed on setting number who knows what, to the tempo of who knows what. The waves of pleasure would rise and feel almost overwhelming, only to dissipate. I got anxious; was I going to orgasm? I tried to stay with the sensation, for over an hour. I even took breaks every twenty minutes or so, as I'd been advised. I didn't get where I so desperately wanted to go—orgasm—even though I know it's about the journey not the destination, etc., etc., etc.

I started to feel uncomfortable, my clitoris agitated and confused. I gave up. The experience reminded me of sexual encounters where I'd come close but hadn't made it, and berated myself for it afterward, for my unwillingness to take up more of my partner's time or communicate my need for a different thing. The truth is, in most of my sexual encounters, I haven't even come close; I've just run out the clock.

Pleasure, it became painfully clear, was a practice I needed more of, and I'm hardly alone. The business of sexual pleasure has swelled into a billion-dollar industry, with companies selling apps, toys, coaching sessions, even THC-infused lubricant that gets your partner high while they eat you out. Sexual wellness brands have flooded Instagram, with Glossier-like styling, many purporting to smash stigma while adhering to a sanitized aesthetic that is explicitly inexplicit. Gwyneth Paltrow's company Goop, for example, now makes vibrators, but don't you worry, they look nothing like vibrators!

"So many vibrators look hypersexualized," she told the *Times* in an interview. "They're either really phallic or they look like something you would buy in a sex shop. I was really intrigued by the idea that this would be something that looked really pretty and cool, and that you could leave it on your nightstand without embarrassing yourself or somebody else." She elaborated, "I think we were just trying to do something… perhaps a little more intellectual."

Are strap-ons not intellectual? Tell that to the millions of people for whom strap-ons are a deeply pleasurable, affirming part of their lives. Are sex shops déclassé, unsophisticated? I don't know, Gwyneth, that still sounds moralizing to me— suggesting it would be embarrassing to have a veiny, lifelike dildo on your bed stand. For some people, that veiny dildo might be a prized piece of décor.

As sexual pleasure becomes more mainstream, as it should, there will inevitably be this calculus of palatability, particularly for entrepreneurs like Paltrow who want to make more accessible something that so, so many people are still not comfortable with.

≠ ≈

There were any number of places I could restart my self-pleasure journey after my failed mindful masturbation attempt. After a wee research spiral I downloaded an app called Kama. It's a new wellness start-up (I know) that aims to transform users' sex lives with educational audio and video content; the free app features exercises to "become a better lover." There are masturbation meditations, sound baths, breath work tutorials, and tips for expanding orgasms, desire, and libido. There's content for both people with vulvas and people with penises; if you're in the latter group you'll find "penetration skills for giving more pleasure" and modules on "harder, longer erections" as well as tutorials for simply "getting it up." What was appealing to me about Kama was its assertion that pleasure is health, and a fundamental human right. Both things are true and underappreciated in our society, but my real question was: *Can this help me relax enough to jack off amid a Chihuahua's panic attack?* That was not covered in the FAQ.

Adhering to "the Kama method," the app aims to help users build new neural pathways that allow for deeper states of relaxation, sensuality, and pleasure. For "vulva bodies," as the app calls them, there are three masturbation meditations with stimulation techniques designed to improve your orgasms, all led by Dr. Saida Desilets, Kama's in-house psychosexual expert. The first was a thirty-three-minute "external pleasure flow" with sound bath. The second was a thirty-one-minute "internal pleasure flow" with sound bath, and the third was a thirty-six-minute guided edging masturbation. The external flows featured touch outside of the vagina that simulated the body's pleasure response, while the internal pleasure flows necessitated finger insertion, with edging a combination of the two. Kama leans heavily on sound baths as a relaxation tool, which immerses the listener in ambient sounds that encourage a meditative state.

Always looking to make things harder for myself, I opted instead to buy a ticket to an upcoming Kama "masturbation meditation" live on Zoom, where Dr. Saida would lead an hour and a half hours of pleasure exploration, an idea that filled me with so much dread I ate a half sleeve of Oreos.

Weeks later, when the event rolled around, I willed myself to have an open mind and a breezy attitude, slipping into what had now become my Maria-is-trying-to-masturbate robe and lighting candles around my bedroom. Saida was joined by Simone Niles, a sound healer and vocalist. The masturbation meditation began with a sound bath as we sunk into our bodies and channeled a meditative headspace. Saida directed us to "smile to our yonis" and to explore, play, and breathe. After some warm-up movements and exercises, we cupped our yonis with one hand and put our hands on our hearts with the other. At one point she encouraged us to locate tension in our bodies and to let it go; I realized my jaw was locked shut, my arms were crossed tightly across my chest, and my brow was furrowed, like a cartoon of an angry person. I tried to release the tension, focusing on my breath and imagining breathing into my vulva. Over the next many minutes Saida demonstrated on her hand a series of motions we were to try on our vulvas. One of the first I found quite appealing—covering our vulvas with one hand, and using the other hand to tap on top of that hand. That woke me right up. But staying with sensation, as we traced our clits and explored our inner lips and vaginal openings with our fingers, I kept snapping out of it—first, to lock eyes with the portrait of Regis Philbin that hangs in my bedroom; then, flipping over only to come face-to-face with my Danny DeVito pillow. After an hour, I closed my laptop.

That evening I talked to Ryan, the thirty-year-old man who has been masturbating the same way since he was thirteen, about mindful masturbation. He was curious but skeptical. After a cursory Google search, he told me it seemed like the technique was more catered to women. Nonetheless, he said he was going to try it. He asked me if I needed any photos or videos for my research and I said, respectfully, no. Please no.

He texted me a few days later. "Per our convo, I went out of my way to make it less of a chore and give myself the kind of love I would give someone else. It was much more enjoyable."

I, however, needed more help. I needed more direction. I needed a coach.

6

I GOT A SEX COACH

"What neuroplasticity really means is that we're rewiring the brain by rewriting our narratives. It's the road to sexual self-realization."

—Dr. Patti Britton, *certified sex coach*

I set my timer to ten minutes and secured my Chihuahua in the bathroom with a bowl of water and a stack of dried pig ears. To run the clock a little, I leaned against my dresser and stretched my quads, wondering if anyone's checked in on Ashlee Simpson lately. I moved toward the bed but then remembered there were Ritz Crackers in my kitchen cabinet due to expire soon. I took care of it. I returned to the bed, caked in cracker dust, and glanced at the timer: 8:34. I could no longer put off my first "homeplay" assignment from my sex coach: for ten minutes, all I had to do was touch my body and explore. There was no objective, no intended outcome, no need, even, to engage with genitals. The assignment was merely to feel sensations in my body. It sounded excruciating.

After interviewing sex coach Amy Weissfeld about masturbation, I realized I could use some professional guidance—specifically, a type of sex coaching that played to her biggest strength and my biggest weakest: self-pleasure. Amid an ongoing global pandemic, sexual partners had become rare for single recluses like myself, so my journey away from bad sex toward fulfilling, satisfying sex would be in my own hands, quite literally. Beyond the social climate, though, it occurred to me that I'd fallen into the same paradox as so many in my generation: optimizing everything in my life—from the amount of overnight oats for maximum energy to amount of boob in selfie for maximum engagement—except sexual pleasure, a vital pillar of sexual wellness. Hustle culture dictates that we grind to get what we want, to become the people we want to be. Even if we resent the premise, we mostly buy into it. When we want abs, we download a fitness app and carve out ten minutes at lunch. When we want to change careers, we grab coffee with mentors and refresh LinkedIn on the toilet. When we feel bad about sex with our girlfriend, however, we simply feel bad about sex with our girlfriend. Or we stumble through a conversation, mostly give up, and bide our time until the breakup.

To be clear: I don't believe everything should be optimized. Some of the best experiences in life are un-optimizable, and call for resisting the capitalist pressure to streamline or upgrade. I don't think, for example, that Gushers can, or should be, improved upon. Fly closer to the sun and you'll get burned. Same goes for wandering around a random park with nowhere to be. You could research better parks, you could research better shoes, but you'll probably just get a headache from looking at your phone.

There are moments when the commodification of sexual wellness troubles me. Any time a corporation profits off people's sexual insecurities, we should tread carefully and critically. And yet, I've found something else to be even more sinister: a widespread learned helplessness about sex. So many millennials I interviewed and surveyed felt miserable about their sex lives, yet had never once considered the possibility of improving it, with or without professional help. The rampant resignation to bad sex, and our ambivalence toward self-pleasure, moved me to write this book in the first place. Pleasure is worth prioritizing, in the same way (if not more than!) we prioritize work and exercise and food and synthetic eyelashes that curl up to our eyebrows. It may not be our fault we have bad relationships with sex—society!!— but no one is coming to help us. We have to work on it ourselves, and outsource guidance as needed.

To insist that people should try to have sex that is less bad, I had to try to have sex that was less bad. To do that, I needed help accessing pleasure in my body, which often feels elusive for the reasons we've discussed: anhedonia (sponsored by my mental illnesses), short attention span (sponsored by my iPhone), and a deep-seated aversion to my body (sponsored by society). Yet again the path forward to better sex, for me at least, was less sex with others. I had work to do on my own, and I tapped Weissfeld to guide me, even though I dreaded learning more about myself. Pleasure is a practice, and I needed someone to force me to practice, because left to my own devices, I would rather do absolutely anything else—even clean the crusty corners of my shower, which is exactly what I did at minute seven of my first homeplay assignment.

"You can't follow the tendrils of pleasure in your body unless you're tuned in," she told me in our first session. "Pleasure is three things: it's attention, awareness that something feels pleasant, and stimulation. In our early conditioning, we hear, 'Don't feel that, or don't go there.' When we talk about self-pleasure, it's [about] paying attention to the sensation in the body stimulus." Relearning tactile pleasure, then, warrants a physical practice, and lots of it. It requires deep, concentrated attention that is not always pleasant.

Weissfeld is a certified somatic sex educator based in Portland, Oregon. According to the Somatic Sex Educators Association (SSEA), somatic sex educators "teach through body experiences," which includes coaching in breath, massage, body awareness, and even erotic trance. Coaches are trained to touch their clients' genitals and anuses "for education, healing, and pleasure," and to foster connection between body and spirit. (Since our sessions would be on Zoom, my privates had an easy out.) Weissfeld is also a "body sex facilitator," meaning she teaches an orgasm workshop, originally devised by the late, great Betty Dodson, famed sexologist and author of the 1974 book *Liberating Masturbation: A Meditation on Self Love*. Dodson, a pioneer in the field of sex coaching and feminist sex theory, recently appeared on an episode of the *Goop* Netflix series, which speaks to the potential of our current sexual moment: you can now see real, close-up, desexualized vulvas on Netflix. And yet.

Weissfeld has shoulder-length strawberry-blond hair and cool, orgasmic mom energy. For our second session, she Zoomed me from inside of a large van, which was never acknowledged. Behind her hung a flag decorated with blue and white abstractions. She spoke slowly and smoothly, like she just came, and her demeanor was casual but nurturing. I realized I would let her touch my genitals if she thought it would be useful. On the other side of the country in Brooklyn, I sat cross-legged on my couch, scraping at the bleached-out portions of cushion where my dog prefers to vomit, only half listening, fearing that if I full-listened I would start crying. I worried that if I slowed down to appreciate all the beautiful things missing from my life—pleasure, playfulness, eroticism—the grief would be too much to bear. We were only exchanging pleasantries and I already felt broken.

To start the session, she asked me if there was anything I needed to feel embodied and comfortable in the present moment. Did I need to change the way I was sitting, or move somewhere else? Was the temperature okay? Did I need a glass of water or a bite of something? Was I hungry, thirsty, cold, uncomfortable? This line of questioning jarred me. I don't ask myself these questions, nor does anyone else, at least not since my Italian grandmother was alive. I fidgeted in my seat, genuinely unsure. I felt numb and sensation-free. Was I uncomfortable? What is uncomfortable . . . Was I hungry? What is hunger . . . I could eat, that much I knew. That much I always knew. I strained to locate hunger in my body but couldn't find it, so no, I wasn't hungry. But I felt a little cold! I think? That tingling on my feet was cold, yes? I counted this as progress—the ability to recognize I was cold. The bar was low. I let my mind run wild with the implications this had on my sex life, which obviously was the point of the exercise: How many times during sex have I not felt right in my body, but ignored the messages my body was giving me? I was on the precipice of spiraling.

"I'm cold," I said, and grabbed a blanket to wrap around my shoulders. I couldn't tell if I was thirsty, so I said I was fine otherwise; I didn't want to waste her time, even though I was paying her and she was begging me to take the time I needed to decide if I was thirsty. Weissfeld has just three rules in her sessions, which, like everything else under the sun, apply to sex: 1. Take care of yourself. 2. Listen to your body. 3. Don't endure.

Don't endure, don't endure, don't endure. Yet again I had been viciously attacked! Enduring is my way of life. It's my heritage, my religion, my lifestyle, my sexual ethos: if something doesn't feel quite right, I wait it out, because that's easier. He's going down on me and I say faster and he goes faster but then he loses the clit and the wave of pleasure dissipates. Well, I've already said my one thing, better now to endure; enduring costs me nothing, or at least costs my partner nothing. What does it cost me?

We began with breath work. She referred to breath as my "inner lover" and invited me to imagine it as such. "It's carrying this nourishing oxygen to all these different parts of your body. It's like giving you a little massage from the inside. It's a nourishing touch."

She asked me to see if I could move my breath any lower in my body. I could not. I couldn't *put* my breath anywhere, aside from sucking it in and barfing it out. I could feel my stomach rise and fall, and the whoosh through my nostrils, but I could not, as requested, send breath to my yoni.

Throughout the session, sex was rarely mentioned. We played a game called "Yes, No, Maybe." Weissfeld asked if she could do certain activities to and with me—give me a massage, go for a hike, borrow $500—and the "container of safety" was that none of these things would happen. For the first round, I had to say yes to everything. The second round, I had to say no to everything. The third round, I had to give my real answer. Before we began, she asked me to gently cup my hand on my vulva, and to place the other hand on my throat or heart. Before and after each question, I was to pause and tap into how my body felt. If I had to say "yes" to something that I wanted to say "no" to ("a hug"), I had to notice what that felt like in my body. If I had to say "no" to something I wanted to say "yes" to ("free money"), I had to notice what that felt like in my body. The idea was to practice interpreting messages from the body, not the head, and notice what it feels like in your body when you say what you want—and how uncomfortable it feels when you don't.

My homework was to enjoy something for fifteen minutes every day. It could be a hot shower or a walk around the block; I just had to notice the sensations with all five senses. I was grateful she backed off self-touch for the time being; that felt too advanced.

"That skill of tuning in to the sensation of the body is known as 'interoception,'" she said. "What has happened to many of us very early in life is that we might say something to a caregiver that reflects a sensation that we feel, like, 'Oh, I feel a tightness in my tummy. I don't want to go to school today.' Right? And somebody along the way says, 'Oh, you're fine, honey. You're just nervous.' When that happens often enough, we learn to translate the sensations that we're feeling in our body to emotions and beliefs and feelings. And we never really reverse-translate.

We never go back to, 'What does it feel like in my body when I feel happy? What does it feel like in my body when I feel anxious?'"

This translation work—surprise—shapes the sex we have. "One of the biggest keys to having good sex," she said, "is the ability to feel that sensation in the body, and to learn how to both expand pleasure, but also follow the pleasure that's there, regardless of how big or small it is."

👁 👁

In the grand, ridiculous history of medical treatment, sex therapy as we know it today is quite new, a small blip on the timeline of human antics. The field originated over half a century ago when William Masters, MD, and Virginia Johnson conducted their pioneering studies on sexuality at Washington University in St. Louis, laying the groundwork for treating "sexual dysfunction." (That clinical term, it should be noted, has become contested. Is one patient's low arousal "dysfunctional," or is her boyfriend simply horrible? Is the inability to orgasm during penis-in-vagina sex "dysfunctional," or is that highly reasonable?) Masters and Johnson developed many methods for treating common sexual problems, primarily among cisgender married couples. To treat premature ejaculation, for example, they employed a method known as the "squeeze technique": you manually stimulate your partner's penis until they are near ejaculation, and then you squeeze three to four inches beneath their glands, eliminating the urge to orgasm. The idea is that the regular practice of the squeeze technique—and another called the "stop and start technique," where you stop stimulation close to orgasm, and then start over—will help the premature ejaculator become more acquainted with the sensations leading to ejaculation, granting them more control over the release.

In their landmark book *Human Sexual Response,* Masters and Johnson shared their findings from studying men and women having sex in a clinical setting, and formally labeled the four stages of sexual arousal: excitement, plateau, orgasm, and resolution. After achieving worldwide fame for their work, they published their second book, *Human Sexual Inadequacy,* which sketched a new sex therapy. Their most influential approach is called sensate focus, which aims to lessen outcome-oriented anxiety around sex and improve communication between partners. Sex therapy with sensate focus is designed to treat couples, wherein one or both partners is struggling with pain during sex, low desire/arousal, or erectile dysfunction.

In a 1970 *Time* cover story featuring the couple, their clinic boasted an 80 percent success rate for treating patients dealing with sexual dysfunction. Masters said, "The great cause of divorce in this country is sexual inadequacy. I would estimate that seventy-five percent of this problem is treated by the psychologist, the social worker, the minister, and the lawyer. Medicine has really not met its responsibility." [1] *Human Sexual Inadequacy* outlines an array of sexual dysfunctions (from premature ejaculation to vaginismus) and psychotherapies to treat them. They claimed overwhelming success in helping their patients achieve greater ejaculatory control, increased intimacy, and reduced pain during sex.

While their work was foundational, their studies' limited

view of sex, concerned primarily with the heterosexual, cisgender sexual experience, means loads of it is useless today. In 1976, researcher Shere Hite, author of *The Hite Report: A Nationwide Study of Female Sexuality,* found that 70 percent of women who cannot orgasm from sexual intercourse can do so easily by masturbation, and became a vocal critic of prevailing sex research and its narrow view of sex. ("Surprisingly, most researchers have not shown much interest in masturbation," she wrote. "Generally, they approach the study of sexuality through intercourse, with masturbation as a sidelight—since, it is argued, the 'sex drive' is fundamentally for purposes of reproduction. However, to take intercourse as the starting point is an assumption—one that has led to widespread misunderstanding of female sexuality.")[2]

Despite their many blind spots, and a horrible book on gay conversion therapy, Masters and Johnson dragged sex therapy into the mainstream. In the decades after, countless strains of treatment for sex-related issues emerged, from traditional psychotherapeutic approaches to a more radical touch-informed somatic practice, in which my sex coach is trained.

Unlike sex coaches, sex therapists are largely barred from touching their patients; they can be psychiatrists, clinical social workers, psychologists, or nurses with specialized training in intimacy issues. In 1973, Helen Singer Kaplan opened the country's first sex therapy clinic, drawing from her experience in psychiatry. She approached "sexual desire disorders" as fundamentally emotional ones that required unpacking psychological experiences like trauma, shame, and insecurity. Much like Masters and Johnson, Kaplan helped usher in a new era of Americans' sexual frankness, which regretfully coincided with increasing sex anxiety. *Should I be having more sex? Should I be more sexually attracted to my husband? Should my dick be harder and last longer?* The more sex infiltrated the public discourse by way of popular media, the more expectations escalated that mind-blowing, multi-orgasmic sex was attainable if you took the correct steps; at least that's what magazines and TV shows suggested. Perfectly timed to play off these fears, Viagra hit the market in 1998, earning Pfizer billions of dollars and transforming the conversation around sex forever: sex was now fully medicalized. In *The Rise of Viagra: How the Little Blue Pill Changed Sex in America,* sociologist Meika Loe writes,

> [B]y 1998 Americans had already begun to transition into a new era in sex, medicine, and technological innovation. Numerous social changes at the end of the twentieth century paved the way for the emergence of a product like Viagra. These changes made it possible for many of us to see ourselves and our sex lives as "dysfunctional." And they began the chain reaction that has resulted in industries and institutions dedicated to what we now call "sexual medicine" and "male enhancement." [3]

And, of course, the social conditions that led to the sexual wellness industry—pharmaceutical deregulation, increasing scientific and popular attention to sex, demographic shifts—didn't impact only men. Women bore the burden to enjoy sex, and to enjoy their partner's medically sustained boner, or to work on themselves until they did. The medicalization of low desire and low arousal pathologizes disinterest in sex—a disinterest that is often quite reasonable. Self-help culture, mixed with this cultural imperative to have a very specific kind of sex, has increasingly put pressure on women to achieve orgasm by doing deep solo work to uncover their deepest desires, and if they can't, "they are also supposed to keep their partners in a state of blissful ignorance (literally) about their truncated or absent pleasure." [4]

This pressure to *love* sex can be enormously overwhelming, and manipulated for profit. This is also true: many people benefit from sex therapy. CBT (cognitive behavioral therapy) has been shown to be effective in treating a wide range of sexual issues, including vaginismus, anorgasmia, and erectile dysfunction.[5] More specifically, mindfulness-based interventions are effective in improving sexual satisfaction among women.[6] Even internet-conducted cognitive behavioral and mindfulness treatments can help women experiencing sexual distress.[7]

Since I already had a therapist (bombshell!), I decided to see a sex coach, both to learn more about the practice and to better understand my sexual dissatisfaction.

There's a lot of overlap between sex therapy and coaching, but some key differences: certified sex therapists tend to approach issues from a more psychological, mental health–focused perspective, and they must obtain certification from the American Association of Sexuality Educators, Counselors, and Therapists (AASECT). Sex coaches tend to approach things more practically, offering a wide range of tools and strategies for improving specific sexual problems. Sex coaching was pioneered by Patti Britton, PhD, a clinical sexologist and educator who popularized talk-based treatment, but there are many approaches. Sexual somatic therapy and sexological body-work practitioners, for example, can stimulate their patients with touch to work through sexual hang-ups (like inability to orgasm or low desire); these more tactile methods have gained global traction but remain illegal in most states, where the sale of erotic touch is criminalized. Sex coaches in general can have a wide range of qualifications, as it's an unregulated title. This can cause some confusion and trepidation, but it also frees up sex coaches to play with less conventional approaches.

"I'm a coach for very deliberate reasons," Britton told me. "I did not want to go into mental health care because I don't believe you assist people in becoming sexually whole or sexually fulfilled as human beings by pathologizing them and by making sex [about] communication disorders or mental health disorders." She avoids viewing sexual problems through the lens of trauma, a trend she feels is too common in the therapeutic world. (For what it's worth, I feel it's not common enough.) While Britton strives to create a safe space for traumatized patients, she finds it much more effective to focus on the present, helping clients "rewrite" their stories to empower and embolden them, rather than dwelling on the same traumatic events. "Of course, there are different ways of being a therapist and doing mental health care, but coaching is so much about the here and now, and moving to where you want to get to. And it's so dynamic and collaborative and interactive."

Even though interest in sex coaching and therapies has surged in recent years, the sexual wellness industry at large remains relatively taboo. Seeking sex therapy is doubly stigmatized for being therapy *and* sex-related. The pleasure-themed episode of

The Goop Lab with Gwyneth Paltrow featuring Betty Dodson marked a promising cultural shift in the popular representation of sexuality, but the framing was still giggly. Dodson's decades-old practice is presented as a sort of novel spectacle—which, for many American viewers, it probably is! Naked women sit in a circle and show each other their vulvas before masturbating together. The show's moments of vulnerability were the most powerful; if we allowed ourselves to be vulnerable about sex, including recognizing when we need help, our pleasure potential would expand. Many women on the show admitted that they'd never looked at their vulvas before, and had seen vulvas (edited, labioplastied, color-corrected) only in porn. The next year, Paltrow debuted a Netflix follow-up series devoted entirely to sex called *Sex, Love, and Goop,* which recruited sexologists to help real-life couples struggling with their sex lives.

We have a long way to go in destigmatizing sex therapy and, frankly, medically accurate sexual information. Pockets of the internet have taken up the cause—sex educators on Instagram post tips and tricks for impact play, pegging, edging, role playing, dirty talking, and other sex acts. While misinformation abounds on social platforms, the sex-therapification of Twitter, TikTok, and Instagram content performs an important role in sharing sex-positive, queer-inclusive information that people are not getting elsewhere. (It should be noted that these social platforms, while doing vital community-building work, remain deeply imperfect: sex workers' and educators' accounts are regularly shadow-banned and deleted.)

A thirty-two-year-old cis bisexual woman, who I'll call Anna, told me she never wants to have sex with her boyfriend again. She also said sex therapy was out of the question.

She remembers the sex being incredible at the beginning of her relationship . . . or was it the same sex as now, filtered through the excitement of newness? Two years in, the idea of having sex with him elicits dread, exhaustion, and that tingling skin crawl of repulsion. Over the past four months, Anna and her boyfriend have had sex one time; her ideal would have been zero times. Though this area of her life is intrusively disappointing, she is opposed to seeking help for it.

"I know this is likely not true, but I feel like talking about it makes it worse," she said. "Like it will make it more stale and contrived, and that it adds more pressure to it. I feel like sex should be intuitive and that you should mesh with someone naturally."

To Anna, the payoff of treatment would be low: she can masturbate "in like two seconds," and she does so every night to go to sleep. She doesn't even desire sex anymore, though she considers herself a sexual person. She concedes that she *could* let her boyfriend go down on her, as a treat for him, but even that would feel like work. "Even still after being with him for so long I'm like, *Ugh, it probably smells. Now I'm taking too long,*" she said. "Even though I know he doesn't care about that stuff."

Seeking help for your romantic life feels awkward at any age, but the unease is especially acute for young people, who believe that sex problems arrive much later in life, when they're married and repulsed by their spouse, or when their penises settle into a perpetual softness. If *Gossip Girl, The O.C.,* and other prestige youth soaps taught us anything, it's that young people be fucking, freely and to completion. The only "dysfunction" is emotional entanglement, never the sex itself. (In the rare instances there is a problem with the sex, it's either traumatic or comedic.)

It took Katie, a twenty-eight-year-old cis straight woman who has been in sex therapy for over a year, nearly a decade to realize she needed help. She's been with her boyfriend for ten years, and she sees herself marrying him in the not-too-distant future, but their sex life was fraught. As a teen, Katie had been in a traumatizing, abusive relationship that made many aspects of sex triggering. She became convinced that something was wrong with her. Having been raised in a somewhat conservative Catholic household, she didn't feel she had the vocabulary or comfort level to talk about sex, which made the notion of sex therapy even scarier. (She recalls a high school science teacher telling her class, "If you have an abortion, you will miscarry every subsequent pregnancy.") Eventually, she and her boyfriend realized there was no alternative; they weren't going to be able to fix their sex life on their own, by sheer willpower.

Once a week, she visits a trauma-informed sex therapist at a nonprofit practice. After over a year of treatment, she can now recognize that her teenage relationship was abusive—and how it warped her relationship to sex. She's also developed a comfort with talking about sex that is invaluable for communicating with her partner. In addition to weekly sex therapy appointments, she now goes to couples therapy once a month with her partner, too.

"We're having sex more often, and it's often better," Katie said. "Though 'better' is nebulous—I more mean we're hooking up and I'm not being triggered by it. I'm so grateful for it."

At the end of each session, her therapist gives her exercises to practice at home; some land, some don't, but they all provide useful information. Because she is sometimes triggered by sudden, surprise touch, it could be triggering when her boyfriend initiated sex, and one exercise helped enormously with this: Katie said to her boyfriend, "Instead of coming in hot, and putting your fingers on my boobs or on my vagina, it's helpful if you start on my knee and push down with a lot of pressure for a while," she told me. "He'll do that for five to ten minutes and slowly try to work his way up. We tried it while we were making out: he puts his hands down at my knee, pressing kind of hard like a massage, and he moves up a little bit at a time. Over ten or fifteen minutes, by the time he was close to where my underwear was, I was experiencing arousal! I felt anticipation that was positive for maybe the first time in my life."

While Katie's sex therapy is primarily individual, it's common for couples to visit a practitioner together. I spoke with one thirty-two-year-old nonbinary person, Alex, who went to a sex therapist with their girlfriend a few years back. Like Katie, their girlfriend had experienced serious trauma that was interfering with their sex life, though Alex hadn't known about the trauma part: all Alex knew was that they were feeling sexually unsatisfied and incompatible with their partner. Alex had a high sex drive, while their girlfriend was demisexual. (According to the Demisexual Resource Center, demisexuals desire sexual activity far more rarely than the general population, and only when there's a strong emotional connection.) Two years in, before they resorted to sex therapy, Alex attempted to break up with her. She talked them out of it. Alex floated the idea of seeking professional sex help, but it took six more months for them to go through with it. The couple saw their therapist for about a year. While the relationship ultimately ended, Alex found the experience illuminating—not only did it improve their sexual openness during the last months of the relationship, but it also shifted Alex's personal relationship with sex itself.

"The biggest takeaway, for me, was devaluing penetrative sex," said Alex. "That was something that was really stressful for her, but it was a stress that she hadn't been able to articulate because, like me, and like so many people in our culture, she saw sex as being first and foremost about PIV [penis-in-vagina] penetration."

During one session, their therapist suggested they take penetration off the table for a few months.

"Because my ex didn't feel worried about it anymore, we were able to enjoy ourselves more and the specter of physical pain and anxiety faded to the point where, when we started experimenting with PIV again several months later, it was a lot easier and more pleasant for us," they said. "Shifting foreplay to the fore was such a necessary and monumental paradigm shift, I think. The realization for me, was that I didn't want PIV—I wanted sexual pleasure and excitement, and I associated those with PIV, but that was a mistaken association that was hindering our ability to genuinely enjoy ourselves in the bedroom."

≈ ≈

At the beginning of our third session, Weissfeld instructed me to put a pillow on my lap, rest my forearms on top of it, and caress it.

I grabbed my waffle pillow, which coincidentally was crusted in another breakfast food (oatmeal), and did as she said. She asked me to lean back into the couch. She did the same. Today she was not in a van, but in a room decorated with artifacts meant to engineer relaxation: a yin-yang placard on the wall, intricate tapestries, a plush couch with pillows that did not appear to be crusted in oats. She wore a loose purple sweater and thick-rimmed glasses with a slight cat's-eye. The pillow she chose for her lap looked fluffy. She began caressing it as I imagine she would a lover. I wanted to know everything about her. I opted to speculate about her life to avoid feeling what it was like to caress a pillow, which was the exercise.

We were to alternate saying things we noticed, "popcorn style." I said I noticed the pillow was soft. She said she noticed her feet on the floor. I said I noticed that the temperature in the room was fine. She noticed her hands were dry. I noticed my dog farted. As we continued, the observations got more specific, the language more precise. I noticed a sort of tingling heat building on my hands as I rubbed it across my pillow. She lifted her pillow to rub the edge in between her fingers. I tried that, too, and felt a soft coolness; I felt different temperatures as the pillow came into contact with different parts of my hand. Just five minutes earlier, my only note had been that the pillow was soft.

Our next exercise was the raisin game. I didn't have raisins. "Oranges are okay," she said. "Or even dark chocolate." I rummaged around my kitchen, laptop in one hand and opening drawers with the other, feeling around all manner of trash in hopes of catching something edible. "Would a loose Peep work?" A loose Peep would not be ideal, she said, but it could work. I rummaged around my kitchen some more and found a slowly rotting apple that still had an edible side. I cut off a slice and returned to the couch.

First, she had me hold it in my hand and say everything I noticed. The slice felt light. It felt smooth. After a minute, she had me touch it; I noticed the softness of the flesh and firm silkiness of the skin. I rubbed my fingers up and down it, alternating the pressure, and then pressed it in between my fingers; the sensation was pleasing. It felt like I was playing on the outskirts of pleasure, somehow, as I molested this apple slice on a video call. It felt good.

The exercise continued with a sight portion (one minute), a smell portion (one minute), and then the most challenging portion: taste, which required I put the slice in my mouth without chewing or swallowing. I agreed and popped it in, but inadvertently began sinking my teeth into the juicy flesh. "Sorry," I said. She forgave me, but I was still tasked with describing the taste. The crunch was louder in my ear, almost like a sound effect. My mouth moistened around the multiplying pieces of flesh as the somewhat grassy, tart, and sweet flecks of juice spread across my tongue. Clearly, all of this was meant to happen on my vulva, if I simply tuned in. My senses were so heightened I'd be very lucky if it did.

When you experience trauma, you often lose the ability of interoception, that capacity to feel things in the body. Shutting down is the body's misguided but well-intentioned effort to protect itself in the face of trauma, and the reflex remains long after the threat is gone.[8] At worst, sex can be triggering for people who've undergone trauma, sexual or otherwise. In better-case scenarios, sex can feel like nothing.

Trauma isn't the only force that takes us out of our bodies. Through early development onward, society instructs us that sexual pleasure is dirty and that our bodies are humiliating. Joseph Kramer, a former Jesuit priest-in-training credited with developing sexological bodywork, opened a school in 1984— the Body Electric School in Oakland—to train others in healing erotic massages and helping patients master embodiment. He believes our society is facing a "plague of disembodiment" that has robbed us of our ability to feel.[9]

Steepening the uphill battle to embodiment are the virtual distractions that erode our capacity to feel present in our bodies, including during sex. Some people fear that porn is propelling youths to over-masturbate and ruining old-fashioned, real-life sex. I'm not interested in pathologizing porn or masturbation, both of which play important roles in healthy sex lives, but as we learned in chapter 3, technology use more broadly does take us out of our bodies, even if we can all agree that electricity is a net good, that the internet is a net good. A 2018 Pew Report surveyed tech experts and academics on the effects of the internet on our well-being; many respondents expressed concern that "online products are designed to tap into people's pleasure centers and create a dependence leading to addiction."[10] Many studies suggest that the negative effects of social media harm young girls more than boys.[11]

The dopamine hits we get from social media are addictive, and the main reason I couldn't complete my next homework assignment, which was to "enjoy something for fifteen minutes."

When I reported this in our session, Weissfeld said I could cut the time down to five minutes. That was my homework, and to continue practicing touch—with any object, not just a pillow. It could be a pen, remote control, or tampon applicator—didn't matter.

The shift didn't happen right away, or dramatically, but over the week I found myself getting more specific about physical sensations. It didn't just feel like "my feet are on the ground." If I truly paid attention, I could notice my soles receiving soft, even pressure pushing upward from the earth. I noticed how temperature and air felt on my skin; how my skin felt on my laptop, typing this. There were little vibrations everywhere. "It's a practice," Weissfeld had told me—feeling things.

In the same way that meditation rewires our neurons to promote a greater sense of peace and well-being, embodiment practices—and, by extension, embodied self-pleasure—strengthen our pathway to pleasure in the body during sex.

Practicing pleasure is a lifelong endeavor, and I resent that to my core. When I committed to the daily awareness practices that Weissfeld assigned me, the payoff was not immediate, but deeply informative. Walking to the Dunkin' Donuts because they had a deal on their gummy little egg wraps, I noticed my arms swaying in the breeze, the cool, dry air grazing them. When I acquired the wraps, I sunk my teeth into the chewy, salty simulacrum of a breakfast taco, and let the gloopy American cheese coat the top of my mouth. In that moment, I could feel and taste everything, and I loved my life. I loved all life, past and present.

A few days later, while having sex with a recurring character, there were moments of gummy little egg wrap bliss. There were moments that felt good all over my body. I noticed these sensations, and tried to sink into them, rather than allow myself to get pulled by any number of distractions: Bucatina licking my toes, my upstairs neighbor's comically loud electric guitar riff, thoughts of climate disaster. But I stayed the course. I remained committed to feeling the subtle waves of pleasure this man's penis provided. After he orgasmed (I hadn't come close), he rolled over onto my arm and removed the condom. I considered asking him if he would go down on me. I wasn't scared to ask—progress—but after taking a few breaths to check in with myself, I realized I didn't want him to get me off. I wanted him to get off *me;* my arm was asleep. I slinked out from under him and went to the bathroom. When I came back, he was already getting dressed. He said he had work early the next morning. I threw on a towel, walked him out, and rushed back to my apartment, skipping every other step. I lubed up my favorite vibrator and lay down on my bed, now gloriously vacant.

I loved my life. I loved all life, past and present.

7

ADVENTURES IN KINK

"[I] implore you to fuck around with dildos, vibrators, strap-on harnesses, anal plugs, anal beads, urethral sounds, gags, blindfolds, or any item at all that you have ever looked at or heard of that has made you go, 'Hmm?' Because only by fucking around with a great variety of implements have I come to my own conclusions about myself. By experimenting with these items, I got in closer touch with what it is exactly I like about sex. And you might, too."

—Eli Sachse in Sex Beyond Gender

When you're a professional sex writer, people assume that you have interesting sexual tastes. Not so. I am a sexually straightforward individual who cycles through the same six positions, the same three dirty sound bites, and, when I'm feeling edgy, the same one request for spanking. I've never had a sexual partner with whom I felt comfortable enough to explore the vast world of kink, nor have I felt moved to explore it on my own while masturbating, because there tend to be more pressing matters: pleading with the dog to stop licking my toes; resisting rumination spirals, laboring to conjure a mental reel of Jason Mantzoukas.

After my sessions with Weissfeld, I realized I needed extra

help with "embodiment," that therapy buzzword signifying something essential, in life and in sex: our ability to be present in our bodies. Countless sex educators and therapists had spoken to me about kink as a tool to access this sense of presence, and I would always nod knowingly, not knowing. People have choked me without my permission, I'd think, but the absence of permission distances this act from kink entirely. Many people in the BDSM community are concerned by the growing misconception that choking is "light BDSM"; sex educator Lola Jean says we're in a "choking epidemic," and most people aren't doing it properly (read: safely, pleasurably). Once again, mass porn illiteracy is making sex worse—and misrepresenting kink.

Most kinky people have an exceedingly sophisticated vocabulary for consent and boundary negotiation; in fact, as kink educator Aoife Murray explained to me, the BDSM community has been decades ahead of mainstream society when it comes to consent, recognizing that it must be ongoing and freely given. This is not how kink is portrayed in most mass media and porn—one of the more flagrant examples being *Fifty Shades of Grey,* a coercive, hardly consensual nightmare wherein the submissive's needs are systemically subdued. Murray, who is a switch, has been a submissive in a relationship with her dom for four years, and wants to push back against the misconception that subs (or any person, in any role) would have to sacrifice their well-being. "Yes, you want to offer submission to your partner if you're a sub, but that's not at the expense of your basic needs. You might prioritize their wants before yours, like, 'Oh, we're going to order takeaway. I might prefer pizza but I think he'd prefer Chinese. We'll get Chinese,' that kind of thing. But this isn't like, 'I need this for my emotional stability but I'll put that to one side.' That's not what we do."

This popular misunderstanding extends to specific acts, as well. (BDSM is an acronym that refers to play that involves bondage, discipline [or domination], sadism [or submission], and masochism.)

"Unfortunately now as BDSM has entered more into the mainstream, there's more BDSM porn and more people going online and finding BDSM, entering it through that kind of lens," said Simone Justice, an internationally renowned BDSM educator and former pro-domme. "Negotiation and consent is one aspect of BDSM that I would love to spread outside of BDSM and into more of sexuality, so that it becomes comfortable and standard for people."

Kink isn't for everyone, nor is it any one thing, but the structure of kink, defined loosely as an unconventional sexual preference or behavior, has allowed many people I interviewed to experience more pleasure, joy, and intimacy, during sex and elsewhere. In addition to providing a framework for negotiating boundaries, kink, and especially BDSM, have been shown to engender a deeper sense of embodiment—the exact thing I, and many of my peers, struggle with.

Simone Justice is among the first fifteen people to be inducted into the BDSM Hall of Fame, and has been active in the BDSM community for over twenty years, mentoring dominatrices, teaching classes, and acting as a consultant for film and TV.

I reached out to Simone because I was interested in working through some of the ways I've learned to leave my body during sex.

She said I came to the right place. The embodiment that BDSM can foster, she said, happens through multiple mechanisms: setting the scene, putting on the collar, using specific language—all are signifiers that trigger a mental shift from stressful real world to fantasy play world. The act of submission, in particular—of relinquishing control, of letting sensual things be done *to* you—allows you to sink more profoundly into sensation.

Simone said that playing with submission lessens the barriers to pleasure—physical restraints, for instance, can inspire a more vivid inner experience. When blindfolds cover your eyes, you rely more heavily on your other senses and feel more deeply in them. ("Our vision is our number one sense, and we over-identify with vision, and we overprocess our vision. When you take that away, people do become much more embodied just automatically," Simone said.) Most important, playing with submission helps you practice receiving pleasure, something that Simone herself has struggled with in the past.

"I can remember when I was receiving, when I was bound and being played with, and having a sense of guilt about it," she said. "I was like, 'Wow, I'm not doing anything right now. I'm just lying here feeling sexy and getting sexy stuff done to me. I'm supposed to be performing and taking care of the other person.'"

Many people I've spoken with, of all genders and sexualities, identified an impulse to caretake during sex, devaluing their own pleasure in service of a partner's. Simone notes that a common misconception about submission is that the sub is powerless—or, if it's a woman sub and male dom, that "they're just following the whole dominant culture thing and they're just submitting to men." In reality, the sub gets to take up space and time and energy with their pleasure.

"In that moment I was telling you about, when I'm bound and I'm receiving and I'm having that guilt of, 'Oh no, I'm supposed to be doing something,' I *can't* do anything, so I'm being constantly reinforced by the bondage," she said. "So I just kind of need to give in and just receive." Regardless of your role in a BDSM scene, the ritual of it facilitates presence, which gives you a fighting chance at embodied pleasure.

The community today is enormously varied, with numerous studies suggesting BDSM's therapeutic benefits among practitioners. Julian Gavino, the model and disability activist, told me that BDSM offered him the freedom and flexibility to exercise control when so much about his life was not controllable. For example, incontinence can be a problem for him during sex, and it used to feel embarrassing for both him and his partner. So, when it sunk in that he could find partners who were into that sexually? Very powerful, and another testament to the way in which kink stretches our sexual imaginations.

Lucy Sweetkill, a professional dominatrix and BDSM educator, learned this in her early years of working as a dominatrix in New York City. She recalls how her exposure to BDSM helped her parse her sexuality outside of work.

"Having that structure with my clients allowed me to have that structure with myself to be like, Hey, what am I interested in? What am I not okay with? When am I not okay with it? When do I want to consent? When do I want to take away consent? When do I want to go faster? When do I want to go slower? When do I want to stop? Filling out that structure for myself was so important and necessary to also understand where in my path did those boundaries not get talked about because we didn't have those structures in place . . . It helped me frame my own internal conversations, as well as then be able to have better external conversations with other people around sex and sexuality and what I want."

Imagine a universe where terms are established before every sexual encounter, and you can change your mind during the sexual encounter, without it being a Thing. While I suppose I intellectually understand why my high school health teacher didn't teach us about BDSM, I would have been much better off learning dungeon etiquette than the location of the vas deferens. If I had learned *any* sort of vocabulary for communicating my boundaries and desires—or even that I had boundaries and desires—I would be a happier, healthier person.

For Sweetkill, her work not only fostered personal sexual discoveries but also opened her eyes to broader social ills: namely, the total lack of education surrounding kink, but also sexual wellness, communication, and consent. She founded La Maison du Rouge with her business partner, Dia Dynasty, in part to help educate clients on kink and sexuality, as well as how to treat sex workers like you would any other professional. ("Would you try to book your therapist or your dentist or your accountant this way?" she said of a late-night email from a client, with the subject line: "any avail??")

Many pro-dommes are similarly generous with their time and expertise, offering workshops, classes, and sessions on BDSM and sexual wellness meant to educate the public—or the small sliver of the public that is willing to learn. Follow them on social media.

Simone Justice is now devoted exclusively to education. After I told her about my struggles with embodiment, she offered to take me to a dungeon in Manhattan for a lesson in domination. She would find a volunteer sub for me to practice on, and I could show up in whatever clothes I wanted to; I could try out whatever I was most comfortable with.

Truthfully, I wasn't comfortable with any of it, but I felt comfortable with Simone, who listened sympathetically as I described my uneasiness receiving pleasure from others, feeling pleasure at all.

A couple weeks before Simone came to town, I got sick (really!) and couldn't meet in person. Instead I perused the internet for classes that might allow me to reap some of the benefits of BDSM; my wish list included confidence, playfulness, and a stronger mind-body connection.

I stumbled upon Mistress Marley's Sexcademy on Patreon. She's a pro-domme and educator who shares resources on her page for sex workers, pro-dommes, and BDSM newcomers. She specializes in femdom and findom, or financial domination, in which the sub's kink is giving money to their dom. She's also the founder of Black Domme Sorority, a collective of Black and Afro-Latinx dommes.

My education began with a video post called "BDSM terms." Most I knew—"impact play" refers to activities involving floggers, whips, and paddles, for example, and "face sitting" refers to face sitting. When she mentioned CBT my ears perked up;

I'm a depressed person (you knew this), and cognitive behavior therapy (CBT) is our bread and butter. She was referring, however, to cock and ball torture, which is a RACK, or risk aware consensual kink.

RACK, like SSC (Safe, Sane, Consensual), is a philosophical framework within BDSM that asserts individuals can consent to riskier acts as long as they're sufficiently informed of the risks.

Murray, the kink educator, goes to college campuses teaching seminars for kink-curious students. One of her most popular sessions is called "Chains, Whips, and Self-Care Tips," and she spends a lot of time talking about risk. When I asked her if she had any suggestions for solo BDSM play, she said, "Whether you are doing it to yourself or another person's doing it to you, you still need to know the risks and be as informed as possible," noting that there are certain activities—anything involving breath play or choking—that solo players should steer away from entirely because they are so high risk.

I still had plenty of options for solo exploration. Murray told me that, during lockdown, a friend of hers taught herself how to rig rope and do "self-ties." I figured I would start even simpler. I ordered a sexy satin blindfold to test Simone Justice's claim that taking away one sense (or more) could enhance feeling in others. The idea made intellectual sense: I often close my eyes before orgasm because I'm so easily distracted by the things I can see. That's why the visuals of porn so rarely move me, because I get sidetracked by details like production value and poetic license. The blindfold would ensure my eyes stayed closed, so I could remain focused on the sensations in my body—while also channeling a little sexiness and novelty because I do not wear blindfolds in my day-to-day goings-on.

At first: panic. I had to remind myself that I could take off the blindfold; there was no lock. It took a few moments for me to settle into the comfort of the restriction, the freedom to stop grasping at total control. As Simone had told me, "As a submissive, you practice experiencing pleasure, and feeling that sense of, 'Oh, I don't have to do anything right now except receive.'" Blacking out my apartment and even the vision of my body, I slipped into a sense of pure expansiveness—my connection to the world hinged only on sensation. Later that day, I wondered if I could ever trust someone enough to put a blindfold on me, given all the sexual nightmares I've endured, nightmares that still live in my body. With the right negotiation, it seemed possible. There's always some fear in pleasure—that if you fully surrender, it cannot be contained. Restraints contain it, encourage surrendering. Maybe I'd try more with a friend.

"There is so much room for platonic play," Murray told me. "It doesn't need to be in a romantic or in a sexual relationship as we've talked about. I could get a new toy and a friend could be like, 'You know what? I've never tried a paddle that's like that before. Would you be comfortable? Can we do a small scene?' Yeah, of course. No problem. I'll happily give you a few strikes with this paddle."

During BDSM play, Murray says she gets a full reprieve from her anxiety. "It's really grounding because you can't fake it till you make it the same way you can in sex. You could try, but you would have a completely unfulfilling experience and it would be so incredibly performative and hard to sustain, because how are you going to pretend that you like being hit by something? You can't. It's not going to work."

She finds BDSM grounding because of its sensory richness, with every prop and garment conveying symbolic significance. When she puts on her collar, she becomes present. Tools are powerful.

8

TOY STORY

"What do you expect, Mother? I'm half machine."
—Buster Bluth

My first time using a sex toy is immortalized in a blog post that earned me twenty-five dollars (before tax) called "I Used a Vibrator for the First Time Today." There are few benefits to mining one's personal life for rent money, but one of them is that the internet acts as a sort of second brain, storing memories I've since repressed because they're humiliating. The downside is that the internet is littered with my most humiliating memories. A later article called "I Wore Vibrating Underwear While Doing My Daily Errands," published as part of my Vice column, Sex Machina, officially cemented my status as person unable to be hired in any other field. While writing Sex Machina, I explored the intersections of sex and technology through a personal lens, writing hard-hitting first-person accounts of using royal wedding–themed sex toys, oral sex–simulating sex toys, and a $2,000 vibrating sex machine called the Cowgirl, which is twenty-five pounds and as big as a torso, with a dildo on top for you to ride.

"In general, people are now more accepting of sex toys," Alicia Sinclair, a sex educator who designed the Cowgirl, told me at the time, in 2018. "I think we're going to see more people investing in larger sex toys, whether it's this one or sex furniture or larger vibrators. Especially folks who are at that point in their sexual timeline asking, 'What else is there? What's next?'"

In my article, I continued, "That's right—vibrators can be unapologetic statement pieces; they can be high-end and luxurious and so, so clearly for sex. A far cry from those looks-like-lipstick or could-just-be-a-ring vibrators; you put the thing on a couch or a bed or the floor, and you ride it, on top of any number of pulsating phallic attachments you adjust to your liking. It looks like a giant, sturdy saddle, atop of which you put the dildo or vibrator. And it's fucking loud."

A few years later, sex tech has become even more ubiquitous. The pandemic and, more specifically, the crushing isolation of quarantine spurred a massive sex toy boom, with brands reporting up to 200 percent increases in sales.[1] But this doesn't necessarily speak to society's comfort level with unapologetically sexual technology. It was still important to Gwyneth Paltrow, for example, that the Goop vibrator she released be "pretty and cool," "intellectual," and not "hypersexualized." Celebrities from Cara Delevingne to Dakota Johnson became outspoken about their sex toy use and signed on to work for their favorite brands—Lora DiCarlo and Maude, respectively. While I enjoy Maude's products, their branding is intentionally, aggressively discreet, with minimalist vibrators shaped like teardrops and lubricant dispensers that are dead ringers for hand soap in fancy restaurant bathrooms, rendering both unidentifiable as sex-related to the untrained eye.

"Despite their growing popularity and widespread use in various biopsychosocial circumstances, many taboos still seem to exist, as indicated by the paucity of scientific literature on the prevalence, application, and effectiveness of sexual devices for therapeutic use," declared a 2021 *Nature* article.[2] Many of the cis men I spoke to said they would never own fleshlights, for example, calling them "sleazy" and "like a less good version of the real thing." The perception seemed to be that owning and using a fleshlight signified a failure to "get" real sex, a deficit that is shameful in a society that constructs masculinity around sexual prowess. (Another roadblock—fleshlights are exceedingly difficult to clean.) I remember, all those years ago, finding my ex-boyfriend's fleshlight on his bed when I broke into his apartment to surprise him. I remember feeling hurt, like his use of sex toys was some kind of betrayal, unable to conceive of someone having a vibrant, full erotic life outside of partnered contexts.

These taboos get in our way. Recent literature suggests that genital vibrators improve sexual satisfaction, both during solo and partnered use, and are effective treatments for erectile dysfunction and anorgasmia.[3, 4] While they can't solve every sexual woe, vibrators and sex tech more broadly are useful tools for exploring our sexualities. If masturbation is the key to better sex, as so many experts suggest, sex toys are the key to better masturbation.

If you're one of the many people who struggles to feel plea-

sure during sex, these devices make it easier to explore and discover the type of touch you love—to be enjoyed alone, and/or
communicated to a partner who, if they can hang, can admin-
ister it on you.

This is not new information; some of the oldest artifacts in
human history are sex toys, which makes our enduring shame
all the more shocking. The first suspected sex toy, an eight-inch-
long stone dildo, was carved roughly thirty thousand years ago.[5]
Hallie Lieberman, who wrote *Buzz: The Stimulating History of
the Sex Toy,* notes that dildos decorated Greek vases and Japa-
nese art. "I think it's important to recognize the history because
it gives a more nuanced view—this isn't a sign of the decline
of civilization," she said in an interview with *The Cut.* "Dildos
have been a part of human culture since the beginning of human culture."[6]

On a sweltering summer evening, I took myself to the
Museum of Sex in New York City to enjoy the industrial air-
conditioning and browse their collection of over fifteen thousand sexual artifacts. Surrounded by tittering friend groups
and couples on third dates, I stood solemn and alone in front
of a "blood circulator" from 1911, a steel crank-like device with a
rubber protrusion designed to treat ailments like gout, rheuma-
tism, and "women's problems" like hysteria and insanity. (The
inventor, G. C. Pulsocon, was imprisoned for fraud a few years
later, but his invention—which produced up to two thousand
vibrations per minute—lived on as a popular underground sex
toy.) I marveled at a jade phallic amulet from the former Roman Empire, the surface of which depicted an unidentifiable
creature performing cunnilingus on a nude woman. To my left,

a man cautiously placed his arm around his date as they gazed upon a contemporary anal plug with horse hair flowing from it, a device I recently learned is used in a fetish called "pony play." I hurried past them, as his date, transfixed by the plug, whispered, "I had no idea." I stopped in front of the Rabbit, the item I'd come to see.

When we talk about the modern era of sex toys it's hard not to mention the one that made it big, that managed to bypass censure and infiltrate mainstream consciousness, ushering in a new era of sexual consumerism. The first iteration of the Rabbit resembles an actual rabbit; it was designed as such to get around Japan's obscenity laws. In 1997, a new model called the Rabbit Habit boasted internal and clitoral stimulation so pleasurable that it earned a role on the first season of *Sex and the City* in 1998. In "The Rabbit and the Hare," Charlotte learns of the Rabbit's wonders and ventures to a sex shop to investigate. ("Oh, it's so cute! I thought it would be scary and weird, but it isn't," she remarks. "It's pink! For girls!")

Carol Queen, the sexologist and activist at San Francisco's legendary sex shop Good Vibrations, declared in a Forbes interview that "*Sex and the City* took vibrators out of the shadows." The day after that episode aired, Queen said she arrived at work to find a line of women waiting outside the store, asking for the Rabbit. *Sex and the City* helped boost demand for higher-end vibrators that people felt comfortable buying inside of a sex store. In the years since, the global sex toy market has swelled to a $33.64 billion industry.[7]

A few cases away from the Rabbit sat Osé, a large, chunky silicone sex device shaped like a flattened C, debuted to the public by sex tech company Lora DiCarlo in 2020. I stood stunned in front of it, mouth agape, and read the little placard. Developed in partnership with the androbotics program at Oregon State University, Osé employs "biomimicry" to imitate "the human motions of the mouth, tongue, and finger by translating them into microrobotic motions." I learned that in 2018, Osé was the first piece of consumer sex tech to be recognized at the annual Consumer Electronics Show (CES) with an Innovation Honoree Award. A month later, CES's parent company retracted the award, calling the product "immoral, obscene, and profane." To reiterate, the year was 2018—two decades after Charlotte bought the Rabbit, and eleven decades after Pulsocon's "blood circulator" gained popularity as an orgasm machine. After a public backlash against the decision, the award was eventually reinstated, and sex toys became permanently allowed at the show. The controversy revealed our enduring discomfort with something as fundamental as sexual pleasure ("immoral, obscene, and profane"!) and, more specifically, the items that help us feel it, typically far more easily than another person could.

My field trip to the museum sparked a deep curiosity in what might come next in the field of sex tech. When I was writing my Sex Machina column, just five years prior, the landscape still felt niche—you found it only if you went looking. (There certainly weren't any celebrities or micro-influencers hawking products.) Nevertheless, I persisted. I tried vibrating vagina Kegel balls, weed-infused lube, ejaculating dildos, vibrating underwear, and an alarm clock–vibrator hybrid that you put in your underpants before going to sleep so you can wake up to an orgasm.

A few days after my visit to the Museum of Sex, on Instagram, the algorithm shepherded me to Cute Little Fuckers, an independent brand that makes gender-inclusive vibrating toys in playful shapes inspired by octopuses, aliens, and starfish, a far cry from the minimalist or explicitly genital-inspired toys you typically find. Founder Step Tranovich, who designs the toys to feel excellent on a wide range of body parts, says the starfish-like toy, called Starsi, has been especially popular with trans-femme people experiencing gender dysphoria—when nestled in the hand, the gently curved toy easily covers genitalia, "allowing us to map new genitalia and euphoria in our own mind." Tranovich, who is disabled, engineers their toys to be held and arranged in numerous ways, so people with limited or no hand use can find pleasure, too. Their whimsical designs also increase what they call "emotional access" to sexual pleasure.

"I had this vision in my mind of someone going to a sex toy store for the first time and going, 'Oh, I don't know. That's too intense,' and then they see my toys," Tranovich said. "It's amazing. I've had lots of people say that [Cute Little Fuckers] was their first sex toy experience.

"The amount of messages we've gotten from people about how the toys didn't just make them feel good, but how important they felt to their gender expression and sexuality and identity . . . ," they continued. "For so many people, these toys aren't just toys."

Another new sex toy start-up called Bump'n has debuted the first line of toys designed expressly for people with hand limitations. The very large Bump'n joystick is meant to be hugged. The company was founded by disability activist Andrew Gurza and Heather Morrison to serve the millions of disabled people around the world who can't masturbate with their hands; their research found that 50 percent of physically disabled people surveyed struggled to achieve sexual pleasure on their own.[8]

🦅 🦅

After gazing upon the Osé locked behind glass, I found the latest model online: Osé 2. Again, I was struck by the device's unapologetic largeness, given the recent trend toward dainty and discreet. I ordered it, and, on a whim, the brand's pluglike prostate/G-spot stimulator, the Tilt, which evenly warms to the temperature of a human body.

As DiCarlo herself is quick to remind you, Osé 2 is not a vibrator (and please don't call it a toy). The round clitoral stimulation end of the device has a hole that you rest atop your glans clitoris, fluttering air to mimic the sensation of stroking and sucking. Because the product is designed for "blended orgasm," inspired by a life-changing one DiCarlo had years ago, you bend the other end to fit inside your vagina, where it simulates a come-hither motion to stimulate your G-spot (the sensitive area a few inches inside the vaginal canal, along the upper wall).

DiCarlo told me over Zoom that her company saw a huge uptick in sales during the pandemic, especially the week the stimulus checks were sent out. "Covid forced us to go, 'Okay, well, I guess I'm going to have to hang out with myself,'" she said. "People realized that there's more to life than just the next social relationship, and that they needed to solidify the relationship they have with themselves. A huge portion of that is sexuality." DiCarlo calls her products tools for self-exploration, in that "they have the ability to teach humans how they like to be touched."

Despite the frequency with which new sex tech companies have emerged—and despite their bids at palatability—these products can still feel intimidating, and some remain in the margins. The fleshlight, for example, has not received the minimalist, cool branding treatment. Designed to mimic the soft, tight canal of a vagina, the device is about as explicitly sexual as it gets. I asked a thirty-year-old cis-het man if he'd ever used a fleshlight, and he responded, "Do I seem like the type?" This reaction was not uncommon.

I asked him to describe the fleshlight-using type. "I would guess it's the kind of person who uses solo sex as a replacement for partnered sex, as opposed to a distinct thing," he said. This sentiment comes up a lot—that masturbating, with sex toys specifically, is something you do when you can't get *real* sex. "I'm not going to rub my dick with a fake vagina because then it's bad sex as opposed to a good kind of entertainment," he said. Using a fleshlight is a less-good approximation of sex, he reasons, so why even try to replicate the real thing? He masturbates with his hands and has zero intention of upgrading. I floated the idea of a butt plug. This, too, was unthinkable to him.

Sex tech can help us discover pleasure in unexplored (or previously off-limits) areas of our bodies, and we can use this information to improve both unsatisfying partnered sex and solo sex. Years ago, I'd tried li'l baby butt plugs a few times while writing my sex column, but I'd never jammed them in deep enough to feel pleasure. I'd also had a somewhat harrowing anal experience with a partner, which is standard when there isn't *lots* of warm-up and *lots* of lube, since the butt famously does not self-lubricate.

The Tilt, the Lora DiCarlo prostate/G-spot stimulator, can go into your butt or vagina. (To find the G-spot, which should more accurately be called the G *area,* DiCarlo recommends using one's fingers to feel around for a spongy walnut texture deep in the vaginal canal.)* The device is the size of a palm and big enough to scare me. When my new products arrived in the mail, I lit some dollar store candles, tucked the Tilt away in a drawer so it couldn't look at me, told Bucatina her mommy was sorry, and grabbed Osé 2, the giant C-shaped robot that would "suck" on my clit on one end and rumble in my vaginal canal on the other.

After lubing it up and bending it to fit my unique "pelvic angle," I sunk into my couch. I took a deep breath, remembering that breath is my inner lover. I took another deep breath, remembering an embarrassing incident from that morning when I mimed curtseying to the mailman after he handed me my *New Yorker.* I turned on the device.

I placed the round head on my clit, adjusting so the small hole would rest atop it. The first thing I thought was wow. The second thing I thought was wowwwwwwwwwwww. The sensation on my clit was distinct from anything I'd ever felt with a

---

* The G-spot, or Gräfenberg spot, is a bit of a hot-button topic. Many experts feel that there is no scientific evidence for this magical erogenous area inside the vagina, though most concede that some people's vaginas have areas of super-sensitivity around where you might label the G-spot. There is no question, however, that the cultural emphasis on this type of orgasm—which is rare for most—has perpetuated feelings of sexual inadequacy.

vibrating toy; in fact, it wasn't vibration at all. As DiCarlo had explained to an unbelieving me, the air-powered motion *was* more like sucking. It felt like the best oral sex I'd never had. Warmed up within seconds, I inserted the other end until it felt snug and turned on the "come-hither" motion. The dual sensations bordered on overwhelming, but were still deeply pleasurable. Its whirring sound marked a stark contrast from the dainty "whisper-quiet" trend in sex toys, and I sort of respected that, even though Bucatina, now taking shelter under the couch, did not. I orgasmed within a few minutes.

I procrastinated using the Tilt. A week passed. The day finally arrived for me to travel to Italy, where I planned to finish this book, so I placed the item in its cute little pouch and packed it in my suitcase, praying that it wouldn't come to life on the plane. Once I arrived at my quaint apartment, nestled in the heart of an ancient Umbrian village, I realized I'd forgotten the lube. *Oops, I can't try it yet,* I thought, doing a bad job of convincing myself that I was disappointed. I peered out my window and watched an elderly woman hang laundry on the balcony of her brick home. *I wonder if this town has lubricant.*

Convinced that experimenting with unfamiliar pleasure points would help me grow as a sexual being, I had no choice but to venture to the town's one supermarket to buy genital gel. Shockingly enough, there was no lube in the personal care corner, just pads and "intimate liquid" for cleaning your vagina. Exhausted by the ordeal of having tried to buy lubricant in a small Italian supermarket, I walked home to rest. Besides, it was 2:30 P.M., national nap time. My hands were tied. I would try the farmacia the next day.

I tried the farmacia the next day. As is custom outside of Italian pharmacies, the windows were plastered with outlandish adverts for anti-cellulite creams, but inside, these stores mean business, stocking a dizzying number of over-the-counter medicines that their pharmacists are extensively trained to assist you with. I kept my eyes down to avoid the helpful interrogation I am used to from Italian pharmacists, which is good when I have confusing diarrhea but not when I'm perusing lubes.

Praise be to Gesù Cristo, there were multiple shelves of sex-related items. Okay, Italy! A boxed bullet vibrator, condoms, a cock ring (?), and . . . gel lubrificante!! Four bottles, all the colors of fruit snacks. I surveyed the options to find one with an ingredient list that began with "aqua," checked out, and rushed home along the cobblestone streets to plug my butt before I lost my nerve.

Back at the apartment, I grabbed a towel from the closet and laid it down on the hard tile floor, making sure my placement was such that I wouldn't lock eyes with my friend across the alleyway, the old woman who didn't know I existed. I considered setting up camp someplace comfortable like the couch or my bed but didn't want to risk dripping lube on the furniture and tanking my Airbnb rating. I had been instructed by numerous sex educators and therapists to use "more lube than you ever thought possible" when experimenting with anal play. I had also been instructed to spend significant time on warm-up. I turned on the Tilt, slathered it in lube until it was dripping, and turned on the warming button to raise its temperature to human body levels, which really did feel like a person's touch against my skin. To continue arousing myself, I activated the external vibrator and pushed my clit onto the "clitoral groove"—think of the device like a T, with one arm of the T longer than the other, which you place on your clit with or without inserting the G-spot/anal stimulator part, the stem of the T. I enjoyed the device as a vibrator, even though periodically re-remembering I was on the floor took me out of the moment from time to time. I squirted even more lube onto the bulbous protrusion, the stem of the T meant for insertion, and eased it on top, not inside, of my anus, which I'd washed Lady Macbeth style in my apartment's old-timey bidet. The vibrations felt good, and I was riding the arousal of clitoral stimulation. As advised, after a few minutes, I turned the Tilt off to try inserting it. Nope. I couldn't push it through. It went a quarter in and my butt said nope. I glanced at the clock: 2:29 P.M. Rather than give up to nap, I caught myself: I'd become laser-focused on one goal, which was to submerge the bulb in my anus. I remembered that pleasure becomes possible when we loosen our grip on expected outcomes and value exploration for exploration's sake. I took a deep breath and let go of my goal. I turned the vibration back on and gave my butt cheeks a massage, gradually moving to my thighs. I put one end of the device on my right nipple until it hardened; I did the same on the left. I massaged my belly button; I massaged my neck; I massaged my kneecaps. And then I took a nap.

~* HOW TO FIND YOUR PERFECT SEX TOY SO GOOD SEX IS NEVER THAT FAR AWAY *~

1. **Browse, browse, browse.** There are many benefits to going to an IRL shop rather than making sex toy purchases

online, the biggest one being that you can get expert advice. Workers at sex toy shops tend to be very knowledgeable of their inventory and can walk you through your best options given your price point and interests. If the idea of strolling into a store and talking about fleshlights makes you uncomfortable, try pretending you are an entirely different person who is not embarrassed by anything. Then, head on inside. Once you're in there, no one is going to judge you! You're all in there!

2. **Stock up on the proper accoutrements.** The full sex toy experience does not begin and end with the toy. To maximize pleasure, you'll want to involve lubrication, as discussed. If you're buying silicone sex toys—which you should, because they're body safe and very comfortable— consider water-based lubricant: it's lightweight, easy to clean, and very soothing on the skin. Oil-based lube will work fine, too, and it's longer lasting, but it's a bit trickier to clean *and* it breaks down latex, so bear that in mind if you, your partner, or the toy itself is wearing a condom. Same rules apply to extra-virgin coconut oil, which is another hydrating lube. Make sure to pick up a good cleanser that you can use after each toy session. Cleanliness is next to godliness is next to staving off infections: sharing sexual devices can increase the risk of sexually transmitted infections. If you're inserting your device into different holes, consider placing a condom on it and changing the condom when you move between holes.

3. **Do your homework.** Before making a purchase, reflect on the kinds of sensations you like the most during

sex or masturbation. (Return to chapter 5 if you feel you have more self-exploring to do.) Is it clitoral, and purely external? Is it vaginal? Is it a combination? Is it prostate? Is it just your nipples? Toys can be mixed and matched—the only limiting factor is price (or potentially allergies to the material). To feel the most confident in your purchase, read online reviews or ask friends for recommendations. If privacy is a concern, and you don't want roommates hearing you, your dream vibrator won't make too much noise. These days, many vibrators are quiet as a mouse; if you don't mind sound, there are also many that are as loud as a vacuum cleaner. Research, research, research. And ask your friends what vibrators they like, now that you've read this whole book and feel super comfortable talking to everyone about sex.

COMMUNICATION 101

"Since many of us were shamed in childhood either in our families of origin or in school settings, a learned pattern of going along with the program and not making a fuss is the course of action we most frequently choose as a way to avoid conflict. As children, conflict was often the setting for put-downs and humiliation, the place where we were shamed. Many of us learned that passivity lessened the possibility of attack."

—*bell hooks*, All About Love

"If I don't like how somebody is going down on me, I don't know how to explain the correction. I don't know how to teach that skill. I think one of the biggest things we're not taught is how to communicate, but men aren't taught how to figure it out either. I would like to be able to explain how to do things right and what I prefer. But even better and more efficient would be for the guy to try and check in with me and see what's working. I've never been with anyone who has done that."

—*Charlotte, cis bi woman, 31*

I t was the night I planned to lose my microvirginity, and I was terrified.

"Microvirginity" is what I came to call a yearlong period of sexlessness, my longest stretch since puberty. While I struggled with the absence of human touch and intimacy, I was mostly grateful for the break. For one, it had freed up more time for creative projects, like making bread one single time. But more powerfully, I sensed a dulling of that bone-deep longing I ordinarily had for sex to fulfill everything—to validate my worth, to boost my serotonin, to tell me I'm pretty. Without sex or harebrained romantic entanglements, I learned to scavenge for these things on my own, providing for myself the best I could. If I felt the urge to text an ex, I sat with that urge, then changed course by FaceTiming a friend: there, a serotonin boost. If I longed for superficial validation, I sat with that urge, then posted a selfie to Instagram Story using a filter that gives you rhinoplasty and cheek fillers: there, some dads called me pretty.

Eventually, the time came to retest sex. With a newfound distaste for bullshit, antics, and shenanigans, I realized I wanted sex, for sex's sake. Anticipating my third date with a guy I liked, set to take place at my home under the pretense of watching a movie, I recognized an opportunity to apply everything I'd learned about myself and my sexuality to the act itself. I was nervous and excited. There would be a human penis inside me, a human penis attached to a human person for whom I had romantic, sexual feelings.

I spent the day tidying my apartment, tracking down loose coins and pills in furniture crevices, shaving my body, worrying—I'd spent half a year researching bad sex. Could I really have sex that was less bad? On the night of the show?

What had become clear to me throughout my research is that the most important determinant of pleasurable, satisfying sex is good communication. It's not even close. You can Kegel every morning and fall asleep to masturbation meditations every night, but if you can't communicate during sex and about sex, you will be disappointed. A lot of us are disappointed.

Indeed, one of life's great tragedies is that other people cannot magically anticipate our desires; they require explicit cues, usually words. But, oh, how we long for them to magically anticipate! How we long for partners to intuit what we want, like sensitive Bill Hader types do in the movies, because that would mean our raw chemistry was so powerful that words were rendered obsolete. From rom-com sex scenes and most porn, we've learned that if people cannot telepathically predict the exact kind of sex we want to have or the exact way we like to be touched, we must be incompatible. We either settle for this, convincing ourselves that sexual compatibility isn't everything in a relationship or a one-night stand, or we don't, jumping ship entirely. There is another, more difficult option, and that is opening a pathway to free and ongoing communication, which requires rejecting the idea of sexual chemistry as a fixed, rigid thing.

"No one's training us how to ask for what we want and need," *Pleasure Activism* author adrienne maree brown told me. "How do we express a no and a yes, those very, very basic tools?"

The payoff of this work—learning to ask for what we want and need—is significant. Couples who communicate about sex—particularly about their concerns—have been shown to have more satisfying sex lives. Communication is associated with better orgasms and greater overall sexual well-being, according to the *Journal of Sex Research*.[1] But good communication pays off only when there's good listening. When do we learn how to listen in bed? We don't.

The unfortunate reality is that without good communicating/good listening between partners, sex will usually be "endured," as my sex coach put it. You will endure (and give) touch that isn't quite right, and you will be too scared, tired, or insecure to say anything. Countless people I spoke with recognized that practicing communication would improve their sex lives, but still couldn't bring themselves to do it—they didn't want to hurt their partner's feelings; they didn't want to ruin the mood; they didn't even know what, exactly, they wanted because enduring sex was all they'd ever known. After dry spelling and sex coaching and masturbation-journeying, I had made a vow to myself: I would never endure sex again just because it felt easier than speaking up.

Cut to the next scene: my date's face is atop my genitals, his tongue scrambling to find the clit. We had been making out on my couch, and he'd just transitioned to oral, a welcome treat. Bucatina wasn't barking (growth!), but rather politely clearing her throat with concern. I took some deep breaths and tried to sink into the sensations I was laboring to feel in my body, just like I'd been practicing. But after less than a minute, he hoisted himself up, moving his dick toward my face.

This is the part where I suck that part, I suppose? I obliged, disappointed that he had been on my parts for just a few seconds, but going along with the program anyway. He grabbed the back of my head, pulling it closer to him. I struggled not to gag. *Okay, this is not ideal. No, this is not ideal . . . But we can do hard things,* I said to myself. The phrase is self-help author Glennon Doyle's life mantra (and podcast title). I've never read her books but the line has circulated Instagram enough for it to rattle around my brain, including during gaggings. Within moments, another competing line began rattling around, this one from my sex coach. *Don't endure.*

I pulled my head back slightly. I continued the sex act, this time able to breathe, and after ten or so minutes, the conflict seemed to resolve itself: he moved to go down on me again. The soft pressure of his tongue felt good. A few seconds later, he stopped—just as abruptly as before—and put on a condom, and we started having penetrative sex. My clit had been just a pit stop, a gesture en route to the main event. I wanted more oral sex, but I felt like I was in a dream where you try to speak but can't. The sex felt nice; I didn't feel like I was "enduring," per se. It was consensual, I was aroused, and the body contact felt thrilling after nearly a year of solitude. But I was settling.

I'd been able to bring so much to the sex that I'd learned from working on this book: more presence, more sensation, and a clearer understanding of what I wanted. But I could not bring myself to communicate. I could not bring myself to ask for what I wanted. This was the final frontier.

Communication is hard! It is hard in general, and it is even harder when genitals are involved. As it turns out, our comfort level talking about our bodies outside of sex is directly correlated with our comfort level talking about our bodies during sex. So, if we're completely uncomfortable with everything, where do we start?

HOW TO TALK ABOUT IT

Beyond the extreme vulnerability of giving and receiving notes during sex, good communication requires energy, which many of us have in short supply. Sensitive conversations feel . . . tedious. But you've made it this far, hopefully I've convinced you that many tedious tasks—like thinking critically about your sex life—are of great urgency and importance. Cultivating a pleasurable, safe, and satisfying sex life matters because the way we feel in our bodies matters. Communication is how we get to good feelings in our bodies when our bodies are with others: we must ask for what we desire, and decline what we do not. (I say all of this with the very big caveat that partners still have the potential to fail us and violate us—more on that later.)

Communicating in general is profoundly difficult, so it follows that communicating naked is, too.

There are two types of sexual communication that affect our enjoyment of sex: a) during, and b) not during. In her research, Pamela Joy, the intimacy and sex coach based in the Bay Area, found that many people don't even feel comfortable talking to their closest friends about sex. Doing so, however, improves overall sexual communication. Since communicating with partners during sex can feel awkward or high-stakes, a good way to build up your comfort level, Joy says, is making a habit of talking about sex outside of sex, with friends.

"It's not quite as loaded as the situation with your partner," she told me. You can take baby steps, too. If chatting with the fellas about your sex life feels intimidating, Joy suggests finding blogs and podcasts on the topic. The key is to practice thinking about sex outside of sex, which makes it easier to talk about sex outside of sex, which makes it easier to talk about sex during sex. A recent wakeup call, for me, was the fact that I couldn't answer my literal gynecologist when she asked me the whereabouts of my yeast infection. I should have been able to proudly say, "Every square centimeter of labia!" Instead I shrugged and nervously smiled, like a creep.

The more you talk casually about sex and sex-adjacent matters, like labia well-being, the more "you eventually find, 'Oh, it's not so scary anymore,'" Joy told me. "I've got confidence with that language. I can say it without being super emotional and more matter of fact."

A recent study found that people's reluctance to communicate about sex is rooted in three perceived "threats": to oneself, to one's partner, and to one's relationship.[2] People are worried that if they ask for what they'd like or communicate what they don't, they could hurt their partner's feelings or damage the relationship, which steepens the potential personal cost. That's why the more comfortable you become talking about sex, the more that feeling of "threat!!" subsides. (What's more, many of us learned to fear confrontation at early ages, often due to gendered expectations—"be a good girl," "boys don't talk about their feelings"—or unsafe/chaotic home lives.) The more experiences you have where communication doesn't end in disaster—"Wow, when I asked her if she could avoid grazing my dick with her teeth, she stopped, and nothing bad happened"—the easier it becomes to speak up.

This was certainly true for Katie, the twenty-eight-year-old woman from the previous chapter who is in sex therapy to improve intimacy with her partner of ten years. She did not grow up talking about sex, and before she started sex therapy, she didn't feel comfortable talking to close friends about it, either. In the two-plus years that she spent working up the courage to seek therapy, she followed a bunch of sex educators' accounts on

Instagram. Consuming this content made her more comfortable with the idea of talking about something that had always felt unspeakable.

"Even if I wasn't totally cool talking about everything yet, seeing that content was like exposure therapy," she said. Gradually, sex felt less off-limits as a topic of discussion.

Whether you're initiating a conversation about pegging at the breakfast table or whispering "no butt, please" during oral, both means of communication require sensitivity and a certain degree of courage. At their very best, intimate acts are delicate dances of reciprocal communication, both verbal and somatic. Sensitivity is required, especially during sex. People are cagey during sex, and with good reason. You are naked with someone, exposing the very genitals and longings society has taught you to fear; that's vulnerable! While I've come to terms with my body insecurities and feel relatively comfortable during sex, there are many things I could tolerate hearing while clothed that I could not tolerate hearing naked.

Nothing is more horrifying to me, a people pleaser, than the perception that I have upset, disappointed, or even mildly inconvenienced someone, and I've built my whole life around avoiding it. The oven in my apartment has had loose rubber somewhere inside of it since the day I moved in, rendering it unusable. For over three years, I could not bring myself to tell my landlord, who is very nice and always available, and potentially bother him to come and fix it. In fact, I have structured my entire life around this unusable appliance—shrinking my minimal counter space with a toaster oven, abandoning baking altogether, cooking only stovetop and microwave foods—

rather than communicate something so straightforward, so neutral. My landlord loves me, and I have to bake cookie dough in four batches because my toaster oven is too small.

In *All About Love,* bell hooks writes, "When we love we can let our hearts speak." hooks emphasizes the role of communication in forging intimacy, something that many of us are socialized to believe we don't deserve. Love is not sex, though they exist in the same cinematic universe, but hooks's framework is useful for thinking about physical intimacy because it, too, is inhibited by the learned sense of unworthiness that compels us to lie or conceal truths. I long for a working oven, but I fear that speaking up might potentially disturb someone. I long to receive oral sex for longer than ten seconds, but I fear that speaking up might potentially disturb someone. I internalize unworthiness, and am left wanting.

These tendencies are particularly common in women and gender-nonconforming people. In her chapter on honesty, hooks remarks that "women are encouraged by sexist socialization to pretend and manipulate, to lie as a way to please." [3]

It's a tale as old as time. The 1993 *Seinfeld* episode "The Mango" resonates so profoundly today that my mouth remained open in a perfect circle of horror during a recent re-watch. While much of the series smacks of the '90s—Elaine's workout clothes, the thrill of fat-free frozen yogurt, pre–cell phone hilarity of airplane pickups—a conversation the group has about orgasms is straight out of the diary I keep meaning to start but never will.

Elaine tells Jerry she faked orgasms during their relationship, when the sex was "enough already" and she just wanted to sleep. To Elaine, faking an orgasm felt easier than saying, "I don't want to have sex anymore." Later, Jerry laments to Kramer, "How did she do it? She's like Meryl Streep this woman. . . . And I had to work the equipment. I'm not unskilled, I'm in the union. If she'd at least told me, maybe I could have done something about it." Kramer admits he has also faked orgasms.

This is the central tension of the faked orgasm, of the drive to please rather than communicate. It obscures or defers a problem (the sex being "enough already") that can be addressed only by a real reckoning with your partner and yourself. But for many people, *still*, decades after the Faked Orgasm Discourse hit the popular consciousness, faking an orgasm is easier, safer, and more accessible than initiating a conversation about what isn't working, even when we're in committed relationships with people we love and trust. Most women who fake orgasms do so, using hooks's language, "as a way to please," an evolutionary phenomenon called "altruistic deceit." [4] (Many types of trout fake orgasms, too.)

A 2019 study found that heterosexual women were more likely to fake orgasms if they believed that their orgasm "was necessary for men's sexual gratification." [5] This is a common belief, because that's the message so many of us internalize from mainstream porn and gender roles in general: sex is for other people's benefit. When you believe this, communication becomes moot. What are you worthy of asking for?

"It's such a huge part of patriarchy, to make your male partner feel like a man, and the responsibility of that is placed on women," Gabrielle Alexa Noel, the author and sex educator, told me. "When you understand masculinity as being able to make me wet and 'come'"—rather than the actual biological machinations of what getting someone wet is—"it's hard to distance yourself from that."

Noel first learned that sex would be for her partner and not for her in . . . church. "I remember being very, very young in church and the pastor suggesting during services that wives need to pleasure their husbands," she said. "And I was looking around like, 'I don't think I should be here. This is church?' That made it hard for me to not lie about orgasming when I wanted sex to be over, especially when having sex I didn't even want to have in the first place." Faking is what happens when communication doesn't feel possible.

The phenomenon has been studied among heterosexual men, who fake during penis-in-vagina sex, too. One study of men aged eighteen to twenty-nine who say they've faked orgasms admitted doing it one out of every four sexual encounters.[6] (Another study comparing hetero men and women found 30 percent of male participants faked orgasms, compared with 67 percent of female participants.)[7] Noel, who is bisexual and polyamorous, started dating women in her late twenties and eventually unlearned the narrow view of sex that made faking orgasms feel compulsory.

But to blame orgasm-fakers for feigning sexual pleasure would be to dismiss the social conditions that make intimate communication feel risky, if not outright dangerous. For many women, trans people, and other groups at disproportionate risk for assault, the threat of violence shadows sexual encounters, disrupting the sense of comfort that communication requires.

We live in a sexually violent culture, and that reasonably affects our willingness to speak up—and to say no.

"It's possible to decide you're going to have sex because that seems like the safest decision to make under the circumstances, and you don't want it to go all the way to being problematic," sex educator Carol Queen told me. "There are plenty of ways society tells people that saying no is not an option."

☙ ❧

A thirty-one-year-old cis woman, who dates both men and women, told me quite frankly, "I'm afraid of men." I'll call her Charlotte. She tells me she rarely communicates during sex. "I always feel very aware of the fact that I could be physically overpowered," she said. "All those experiences of being pushed through something that I don't want to do has increased the fear."

Agreeing to sex you don't want to have is not the same as faking an orgasm, but the objective is often similar: to placate or please a partner, because that feels safer. Even when there is no obvious threat, many people are hypervigilant about their partner's experience at the cost of their own.

Hailey Magee, the codependency recovery coach, calls this behavior "sexual people-pleasing." Magee helps her clients learn to set boundaries and communicate authentically, rather than contorting themselves for external validation. Codependency is a learned emotional and behavioral condition that affects someone's ability to form mutually satisfying relationships.

Codependent people often have low self-esteem and "look for anything outside of themselves to make them feel better," according to Mental Health America.[8] As Tian Dayton, PhD, describes it, "Codependency is fear-based and is a predictable set of qualities and behaviors that grow out of feeling anxious—and therefore hypervigilant—in our intimate relationships."

These traits often develop gradually as the result of childhood trauma, but not always. Many of us learn to people-please by Living in a Society where we're asked to suppress our own needs to stay safe (or even simply to remain desirable—which can feel like safety).

"I need to be liked," Charlotte, who identifies as codependent, told me. "I don't want to make the other person feel bad that I'm not having a good time. I'm also so used to my pleasure not being the priority; it hasn't been important enough for me to want to overcome those things. I've been noncommunicative for a while and I will continue to be."

Codependent people feel that telling the truth about their feelings would threaten their safety or well-being. Magee says that common confessions among clients of all genders who struggle with communicating during sex include "I didn't really want to, but I didn't know how to say no, so I said yes instead"; "It was just one orgasm. He'll never know it wasn't real"; and "It's hard for me to receive pleasure. I don't know why. It just is."

"When we participate in unwanted but consensual sex, it isn't necessarily obvious to our partners that we aren't enjoying ourselves," Magee writes. "After all, people-pleasers have this down to a science: feeling one way, but acting another. We are among the world's greatest performers."

Charlotte says her mentality during unpleasant sex is to wait it out. "I'm not very comfortable asking for something that's not happening or saying that I don't like it," she said. If there's a hand somewhere she doesn't want it to be, she usually can work up the chutzpah to move it. But anything beyond that feels too intimidating. In general, she is extremely uncomfortable talking about sex. She blames her childhood. "I was homeschooled, so I was very much taught nothing," she said. "My lovely mother who I love very much had so many misguided ideas. She sat me down when I was a teen and said, 'If you give oral sex, you're a prostitute.' I feel like every sexual encounter I have is laced with shame—before, during, and after."

Beyond fear and shame, which so often present as codependent-like behaviors, there are other deterrents to communicating. A common one is the idea that talking about sex breaks the spell. A thirty-one-year-old cis bi woman I spoke with, who I'll call Rebecca, fears that communicating "will ruin the moment and become less sexy. Also a few times when I did try to correct my partner, the change wasn't any better, so I definitely didn't want to correct a second time."

Rebecca's trepidations about communication hinge on three common assumptions: 1. Communication is not sexy. 2. Communication isn't worth the trouble, especially if you're not sure what you want. 3. Communication could hurt your partner's feelings.

I'll start with number two. True communication requires knowing what you want—or what works—which can be the trickiest part. I find Emily Nagoski's *Come as You Are Workbook: A Practical Guide to the Science of Sex* to be an extremely helpful tool for gaining a greater understanding of your relationship to desire, pleasure, and arousal (three very different things, by the way). For people with vulvas, Laurie Mintz's *Becoming Cliterate: Why Orgasm Equality Matters—and How to Get It* is a useful resource as well. Exploring your body outside of partnered contexts is typically where the discoveries happen, when there's no one else to please or perform for. That's part of the reason why developing a masturbation practice is so rewarding; in what other context would you feel comfortable enough to insert a vibrating butt plug for the first time? In front of an audience? Maybe you're into that kind of thing. But maybe not. If you find you love the butt plug—which I think you will—you can then relay this information to partners. And this principle transcends butt plugs. Other insights you might only learn alone could be, "I can only come when fingers circle around my clit counterclockwise," or "I think it would be hot if you pretended to be the mailman," or "I'd prefer if you stopped pretending to be the mailman, I don't understand the scene."

As for Rebecca's first concern—that communicating during sex ruins the mood—she corrected herself a few hours after we spoke, sending me a video she'd filmed of her laptop screen: Samantha from *Sex and the City* is naked and sitting on a naked man. She gently instructs him how to stimulate her clit, interspersed with breathy sounds of pleasure and physical reinforcement. "Now put your index finger on my clit . . . Good . . . little less pressure . . . Ooohkay now two fingers." She grabs his head and kisses him on the lips. "A little higher . . . A little bit more to the left . . ."

"Well, Samantha makes communicating during sex look sexy," Rebecca texted.

Rebecca's reluctance to communicate multiple times during sex came from a fear it would disrupt the flow and be too much trouble. In this brief clip, Samantha communicated six instructions, and the scene was still hot, sexy, flowy.

So what *should* we be talking about during sex? Well, all the things Samantha said, things like "faster," "slower," "harder," "counterclockwise," "just like that," but also things like "I'm tired," "Do you like that?" "I have to pee." Once we've done the work to figure out the kind of touch we love, we owe it to ourselves to bring that to partnered sex, and to seek out sexual situations—casual or otherwise—where we feel safe enough to communicate.

We can also recruit tools from the world of kink, including the traffic light system, which simplifies mid-play communication to one word, with no further explanation required. Aoife Murray, the kink educator, told me she uses a traffic light system to communicate: green (love this, let's keep going), yellow (let's pause, I need a glass of water), red (hard stop), and blue, which Murray might use if she's experiencing anxiety and doesn't know what she needs.

"Saying no requires no justifications," she said. "It's really common that we try and wrap up our consent in this pretty little bow. And we say, 'Would you mind not doing that please?' And we start with the explanation like we're writing someone an essay. In BDSM, you go safe word first and then if it feels appropriate and it feels safe to do so, explanation afterward."

Not only is the online series OMGYes a smart resource for masturbation inspiration, but it offers a master class in communication: at the end of each video, there's an interactive feature where you stimulate the woman's clitoris with your cursor, using the technique detailed. If you're doing it well, they tell you something like, "Just like that." If you need to be redirected, they might say something like, "A little faster." Even in the instances where I failed to stimulate the virtual clit in the way the computer woman wanted, her feedback was always positively framed, and offered in an encouraging tone:

"Slow for now is good."

"Just above my clit."

"Even faster."

"I like that."

"Hello, is anybody there?" (She said this when I took a break to refresh Instagram.)

As for Rebecca's third concern, about hurting her partner's feelings, well, he may just need to learn how to listen.

LISTENING ABOUT IT

Not too long after I lost my microvirginity, I had another opportunity to practice communicating in bed. After a few pleasant dates, I invited a man home. As Bucatina paced around the apartment, licking my toes whenever they jutted off the bed, the man and I bounced around between sex acts, none of them quite working for either of us. At one point, he began to play with my clit. "Do you like that?" he asked. "Yes," I said. My breathing got heavier; my legs periodically stiffened as the sensation spread through my body. At one point, the pressure of his fingers became a bit too intense. My first instinct, rather than say anything, was to try getting used to it, to undermine the sensations in my body. My body, however, ratted me out; this partner, intuitive and compassionate, could tell that I was no longer enjoying it. The little pleasure sounds had stopped, and my legs had softened, laying still, as I thought about breakfast. He asked, "Is this good?" That tiny three-word lifeboat made it easy for me to say, "A little softer." He softened his touch, and we were back on track. "A little faster," I added. We were even further down the track.

Our sexual partners will not always toss us tiny lifeboats. Most of us receive little to no modeling of healthy sexual communication, so we have to work at it—both speaking and listening. We cannot count on our partners to be good listeners, but we can practice being good listeners ourselves. We can make sure we're never the person who cruises past signals from our partners that something doesn't feel good.

Studies have shown that in heterosexual encounters, men overestimate women's interest in them, and it's this precise genre of delusion that exacerbates the bad-listening problem. (From a psychological perspective, if you perceive a situation to be one way, you likely won't hear evidence that contradicts your perception—a phenomenon known as "filtering.") Abandoning assumptions before, during, and after sex makes you a more receptive, empathetic sexual partner, one who becomes capable of making their partners feel good. We need to populate the world with more of those people.

First and foremost, good listening is "active listening," a term coined in 1957 by American psychologists Carl Rogers and Richard Farson. It remains one of the best technical frameworks for listening well, as it requires observing nonverbal cues and fully digesting verbal ones, then paraphrasing them back to the speaker. The three main steps of active listening are comprehending, retaining, and responding, and all three are fundamental to pleasurable sex. While paraphrasing back during sex might seem like overkill, it's worth giving a chance. "Paraphrasing back in the middle of sex is hot as hell and I'm actually not sorry," a friend told me when I asked her opinion. "But also, paraphrasing back can look like reading the room and being like, 'Oh you like that, don't you.' It's not necessarily a Power-Point or whatever."

During sex, it's not uncommon for people to miss all three steps. Example: the men who've spent too much time on my nipples did not *comprehend* I was so bored with the sex that I was mentally reciting the fifty digits of pi I have committed to memory. Then again, they had nothing to *retain* or *respond* to: I was mentally reciting the fifty digits of pi I have committed to memory. I didn't speak up, and they weren't mind readers.

That's why active listening is a useful place to start, but it needs to be tweaked for the peculiarities of sex and our hang-ups about it. Consent educators are doing some of the best work around intimate communication. While consent is a limited framework for modeling reciprocal, pleasurable sex—you can consent to sex that sucks, and we're trying to raise the bar here—it's a necessary place to start. Sarah Casper is a consent educator who works with children, parents, and schools to teach communication. Casper, who posts educational videos on her Instagram account @comprehensiveconsent, has her reservations about the word "consent," too; she basically uses it as shorthand for so much more. "Consent is a legal term," she told me. "We tend to also use it in non-legal settings instead of words like 'boundary' or 'permission' or 'agreement.'" She teaches boundary-making, decision-making, and the principles of bodily autonomy, with the goal of equipping kids and teens the skills "to practice consent in low-level everyday settings, so that they're prepared for relationships in the future."

Casper, who has a background in psychology, practiced partner acrobatics for years, which helped her develop a vocabulary around communication. To collaborate successfully with another person in highly vulnerable contortions, wherein a wrong move could shatter a skeleton, you needed much more than consent or permission—you needed active, ongoing communication. She realized that communicating about the body was bigger than sex—it could be practiced in just about every area of life. There was never a "right" or "wrong" way for two bodies to interact, she found—there was merely a "yes or no *right now.*" Context was everything. If you assumed something was okay with your partner, something that wasn't mutually and constantly negotiated (say, that they would be the flyer, because they were smaller), someone could get their neck snapped. When I talk about moving beyond active listening, which requires someone to say something first, I'm talking about checking in.

"Checking in is something that's just not talked about," Casper said. In conversations surrounding consent, "the question is always, 'Did you get a yes?' or even, 'Is that okay?' That's a very different check-in than, 'How would you like me to touch you right now?'"

Checking in is good listening. The more specific the check in, the better. People want to be touched in different ways in different scenarios, in different places, with different people. That's why communication needs to be ongoing, and check ins should cover whos, whats, wheres, whys, hows, and whens. To make her point, Casper described an imaginary child who hates getting long, wet kisses from his mom at school. If the child can figure out not just *who* he wants kisses from, but when and where and how he wants kisses at all, he can communicate this boundary clearly to his mom. "[The framework] helps you break down, 'Oh, I like kisses from Mom, just not at school.' As opposed to, 'Mom, I don't like when you kiss me, period.' It also helps decenter the 'who,' because he's saying, 'Mom, I don't want *anyone* kissing me at school.'" Decentering the who helps with the whole "But what if I hurt their feelings?" problem.

Casper draws inspiration from longtime therapist and sex educator Betty Martin, who created "The Wheel of Consent" to help illustrate the dynamics of human interaction. The wheel is divided into four quadrants—there are two questions, asked by two people, creating four possible interactions. One exercise for practicing consent between two people involves Partner One asking, "How would you like to touch me?" Partner Two says what would feel good, and if Partner One agrees, Partner Two offers this type of touch—for his benefit. Partner One then asks, "How would you like to be touched by me?" Partner Two shares what would be the most pleasurable for him, and if Partner One agrees, he touches him in this way. Then they switch roles and repeat the questions. The idea behind the wheel is to a) understand the four potential dynamics of a sexual interaction, and b) to get hyper-specific about what you want, knowing that you can change your mind at any moment and so can your partner. (The diagram below is adapted from The Wheel of Consent, © Dr. Betty Martin.)

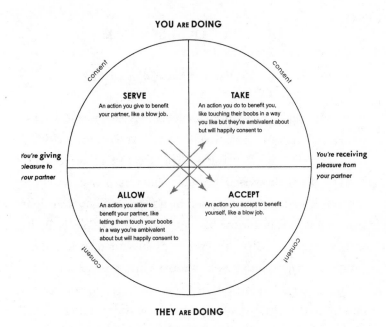

The exercise is all about getting comfortable with receiving pleasure for your own sake, not someone else's, and also with giving pleasure for the sake of your partner's, not your own. Each of these mini conversations requires active listening: comprehending, retaining, and responding. The Wheel of Consent is designed to help people surrender wholly to pleasure, within the safe container of consent. As Martin writes in *The Art of*

Giving and Receiving, "The one factor underlying whether we can enjoy being touched, in any way at all, is knowing that we have a choice in the matter.... If you attend to the process of noticing what you want and communicating, the quality of your experience vastly improves."[9]

TIPS FOR GOOD SEX TALK

1. TALK ABOUT SEX OUTSIDE OF SEX

Pamela Joy, the sex and intimacy coach, suggests forming a discussion group with close friends to talk about sex. She offers a free resource on her website called "Down to There Circles" that proposes discussion prompts, questions, and resources for weekly gatherings, in-person or virtual, with four to eight friends. Her theme for the first meeting, for example, is myths surrounding sexuality. She poses discussion questions like, "What messages did you receive as a child around sexuality? In the home, in the world?"; "What messages do you receive now? How do these impact your sex life today?"; and "What messages would support a healthier relationship with your body and sexuality?"

Listening to sexuality-themed podcasts is another way to develop a comfort level surrounding taboo conversations. I like SexualiTea, hosted by a certified sex therapist (Mia) and a sex and kink educator (Kia), and Better in Bed, hosted by sex coach Sara Tang. Consuming sex-positive content from Instagram sex educators can help build your vocabulary, too. Eva Bloom

(@whatsmybodydoing), Yana Tallon-Hicks (@the_vspot), Portia Brown, Gabrielle Smith, and Gabrielle Kassel are a few of my favorite creators in that space.

Eventually, you're likely to become more comfortable talking to your sexual partners about sex in daily life. One comfy place to start is with meta-communication—communicating about communication. An example: "I would like to talk to you about something, but I'm feeling kind of nervous about it." If you're scared your partner will feel criticized, share that. Vulnerability is not the enemy. Try to initiate uneasy conversations in spaces where you both feel comfortable, like in front of the *Puppy Bowl.*

If you don't tend to have regular partners where there would be regular opportunities to talk about sex outside of sex, be brave and create those opportunities. Make the most of those awkward fifteen minutes when you bring your date back to your place and just sort of stare at the ground in silence before making out. Recruit inanimate conversation pieces to help you—sometimes I'll leave a vibrator out on the coffee table before going on a date, so if we return, I can be like, "Oops, how did this get here!!" This is a good segue into, "I love my vibrator," which is a good segue into using it during partnered sex—something I love, but am not always comfortable asking for during the act. Sharing sexual fantasies outside of sex is a great way to lower the stakes and plant the seeds for future experiences.

If you're still terrified of "kitchen-table sex talks," i.e., sex talks in casual settings—a term first coined in Dr. Laurie Mintz's excellent *A Tired Woman's Guide to Passionate Sex*—

check out mojoupgrade.com. It's a quiz designed to help couples communicate their fantasies. "We spare you the fear of embarrassment by ensuring that we only show you the questions where you both have indicated a willingness, not those where one or both of you said 'no.'"

Another communication lifeline you can throw yourself in advance of an expected sexual encounter, Magee (the codependency coach) suggests, is setting boundaries ahead of time, even over text—say, "Let's keep things friendly tonight, and if there's chemistry, we can do more another time." [10] Or perhaps you're stressed about something else, like how long it takes you to orgasm. You could say beforehand, or during the make-out stage, "Just so you know, I don't usually orgasm during sex," and that might help take some of the pressure off. Working with a sex therapist or coach is another way to practice sexual scripts that you struggle with in the moment.

2. OUTSOURCE INSPIRATION

To communicate well in bed, we first must deprogram some of the toxic messages we've spent our lives internalizing: namely, that passionate sex is wordless and that good sexual partners intuitively know what we want. We learned these messages through media, and we can unlearn them through media as well. OMGYes videos and ethically made, feminist, and queer porn offer wonderfully vivid inspiration for how to kindly direct somebody during sex and course-correct when you want something different. Dipsea is an app that's basically audio porn, featuring inclusive and sex-positive stories that turn you on and offer inspiration.

Practicing communication and consent also helps minimize some of the sting we ordinarily attach with yeses and nos. We can take inspiration from the BDSM community, where setting boundaries isn't a rebuke, but a requirement.

"My definition of domming is creating a space where someone feels comfortable enough to be at their most vulnerable and competent enough to advocate for themselves," pro-domme and sex educator Lola Jean told me. "Yeses and nos aren't successes and failures, just information. We attach emotion to a lot of these things when our partner says something like, 'I'm not having a good time.'"

Pro-dommes are among the best sex educators out there, and many educators in the BDSM community offer online resources, videos, and tutorials that deal with effectively communicating in sexual contexts, a big part of which is boundary-setting. Lindsay Goldwert's book, *Bow Down: Lessons from Dominatrixes on How to Get Everything You Want,* is a fantastic resource as well.

Lucy Sweetkill, the New York–based pro-domme and sex educator, told me that the structure of BDSM offered her the tools to negotiate her sexual desires and have sex that was truly fulfilling. BDSM, and sex work more broadly, requires negotiation long before anything sexual happens—and the negotiation is ongoing. In advance of sessions, Sweetkill's clients fill out extensive questionnaires on their likes, dislikes, desires, and hard nos. She reviews these answers a second time when her clients arrive in person.

"It's time to confirm, 'Hey, you wrote these things. You said you're interested in these things. You meant that, right? And here are the things you say about your limits and your boundaries. You meant that, right?'" she told me. "You create this process where negotiation is very important, and conversations have to be had before you even start anything. People need to agree with what possibly can happen. And when we end our scene, we know we ended and what we expect to happen afterward. Having it totally broken down into all these steps is something we don't do in regular life when it comes to relationships and sex. There's so much place for miscommunication and assumptions and stuff getting messed up in the messaging."

3. PRACTICE, PRACTICE, PRACTICE

"It takes time and repetition to be a good communicator," Sarah Casper told me. "It's really hard to get that when you're an adult. I still make mistakes, but I like to think that I make less than I did three years ago."

Part of being a good communicator is being a good listener. Don't assume that you know what your partner wants without checking in with them; reject the myth that asking your partner what they want makes sex less sexy. Practice active listening in every part of your life, and practice giving your partner opportunities to speak up, by asking "Does this feel good for you?"

To keep conversations productive, Laurie Mintz recommends starting sentences with "I" rather than "you," which can come off as accusatory. "Contrast how you would react if your partner said 'You never go down on me!' with 'I'd love you to go down on me more often,'" she said. "My guess is that the 'you' statement would result in you feeling attacked, defensive, or guilty. The 'I' statement, on the other hand, would hopefully be an entry into constructive dialogue." [11]

If full sentences feel like too much, practice these words: "Faster." "Slower." "Harder." "Softer." "Yes." "No." "Ouch." "Wrong hole."

To build confidence communicating outside of sexual contexts, Martin's *The Art of Receiving and Giving* offers numerous low-stakes, sex-free exercises. One such exercise is the "Three Minute Game," first developed by Harry Faddis, that I described earlier in the chapter. It requires two people who take turns asking two questions—"How do you want me to touch you for three minutes?" and "How do you want to touch me for three minutes?"—and the other person does the agreed-upon action for three minutes, only if they are willing. "When your partner asks what you want, pause to notice what sounds wonderful. Ask for it as directly as you can," writes Martin. "When you ask your partner what they want and they tell you, pause again and notice, 'Is this a gift I can give with a full heart?' Set limits as needed."

For those of us who mostly have sex with people we meet on the internet, these tools are a little more challenging to practice, but not impossible. I am blown away (the good kind) when someone asks me, "Can I kiss you?" after a successful date. The real challenge will be—and this hasn't happened yet—when someone asks me and the answer is no. (Usually when someone wants to kiss me who I don't want to kiss, my body language is so severe they don't bother trying.) I'm playing out such a scene in my head, where someone asks and I don't want to, and my instinct is to lie, even in this low-stakes brain scenario—anything but say no, I don't want to. ("My doctor hasn't actually cleared me to kiss right now.") Something I recently learned in a therapy program is that lying is actually bad. When we lie to "protect" another person's feelings, we send a message to ourselves that our authentic needs, desires, and values are not important. Authentic communication builds self-esteem. Self-esteem builds better sex lives. The prosecution rests its case.

CONCLUSION

"Pleasure lets you make friends with your body, and that changes your sense of who you are in the world, and your sense of self-worth, value, and compassion. Many fears and inner conflicts resolve. That is why it is often said that pleasure is our primary healing modality."

—Dr. Betty Martin

Loitering in the parking lot after a long, humiliating day of middle school, my friends and I were riding the sugar high of vending machine Pop-Tarts. Most of us were a year or so away from seriously counting calories and structuring our worth around smallness, so the two "blueberry" toaster "strudels" inside the silver packet went down easy. Field hockey practice didn't start for another half hour so we walked lazily to the field, gossiping and making fun of one another's biggest insecurities. It wasn't too long before the conversation turned to crushes and romance, as it is wont to do when preteens have too much idle time. One girl named Claire announced that someone in our peripheral circle had given a boy a hand job. Now, I'd heard tell of *blow* jobs. The delinquent boys were always snickering about them in the back of the classroom, cataloging the girls in our grade who'd given them or were most likely to. Not knowing a single thing about dicks aside from their capacity to urinate, blow jobs didn't add up to me—I wondered whether the sucking was for the benefit of the mouth or the penis—but at least I understood the general mechanics. When Claire mentioned hand jobs in the parking lot, though, I was out of my depth. What the hell? I was stumped, even though the name of the act essentially describes it.

"Why would you suck on a guy's fingers?" I asked. It was so inconceivable to me that people felt pleasure on their penises, that genitals were where we felt pleasure, or that sex acts had anything to do with pleasure at all. To me this ever-growing number of sexual maneuvers I was expected to know were entirely random: roll die for first body part, roll die for the second, make them interact. Tell your friends about it. Repeat.

I could label fallopian tubes on a worksheet, I could even explain how a diaphragm worked, but I could not tell you why we had sex—not during my vending machine Pop-Tart–eating days, and not even during my first several years of sexual activity.

The girls should have laughed me out of town for that question; I should have had to change schools. God must have smiled down on me that day. "It's when you rub your hand up and down on a boy's penis," Claire corrected matter-of-factly. "Oh right," I said, kicking my field hockey stick and catching it above my shoulder. "I know that one."

All of sex felt scary to me, even the fringe acts. At no point during middle school and high school sex education classes did it become clear to me why humans engaged in this clearly life-ruining activity. I was so adept at absorbing our culture's cis-heteronormative, fear-based messaging around sexual health that I didn't explore sexual pleasure on my own, not even in private, until college, and my relationship with it remained fraught for years to come. When I eventually became sexually active, I found sex to be fun, interesting, and validating. Hooking up became a novel way to pass the time and generate brunch conversations. The sex, though, was almost universally unsatisfying. I didn't mind, and I don't blame myself now. Looking back, I wonder what my sexual history would have looked like if I'd learned that sex was supposed to feel good, if I had learned this in school or at home or in the parking lot before field hockey. Would I have tolerated—nay, sought out!—all that bad sex? Would I have found deeper romantic fulfillment? Would I have found it easier to say no? In my thirty-one years on Beyoncé's earth, I have never needed to identify fallopian tubes on a worksheet, even though my sixth-grade health teacher gave me the impression this would come up constantly. What has come up constantly is bad sex.

What makes bad sex so bad, or worse than any other bad thing? Is sex a big deal? Is it *a* deal? Is it more meaningful, more special than other physical interactions, like handshakes or hugs? If you're religious, your answers to those questions might be yes. If the society you live in is shaped by religious ideals, your answers to those questions might be yes. Those answers—and anyone's personal relationship with sex—is valid. But can we explain why sex is special without relying on belief systems? Are we—am I—justified in demanding more of sex than we demand of other activities? I get bad haircuts all the time, and yet I'm not moved to write a book about it (though maybe that's what it will take for my stylist to stop gaslighting me into blunt bobs).

The question of sex's "specialness" stumps legal scholars, too. In the eyes of the law, sexual assault is considered worse than nonsexual physical assault. A sexual violation is considered more damaging than other violations—why? I agree that it is, but exceptionalizing sex can get us into trouble, too. The criminalization of sex work assumes that the exchange of sex is fundamentally different from other exchanges, and this harms sex workers by making it harder for them to organize, migrate, access health resources, and find socioeconomic security. The stigmatization of sex work and this belief that sex is special— more special than gas-pumping or tax-filing or toilet-fixing— marginalizes workers and leaves them more vulnerable to exploitation.

Indeed, the law can't tell us what sex means, nor is it equipped to fully define sexual justice. Therefore, we must collectively imagine a framework for sexual justice that's bigger than consent, a limiting legal term. Especially when we're talking about bad sex, which is all I ever talk about. I have spent a lifetime consenting to bad sex; does that mean all is well and good in Marialand? In *Screw Consent: A Better Politics of Sexual Justice,* Joseph J. Fischel writes, "Bad sex, even if consensual, can be really bad, and usually worse for women: not just uninspired, unenthusiastic, or boring, but unwanted, unpleasant, and painful. That problem cannot be addressed by consent. Worse still, the problem of bad-as-in-really-bad sex is automatically deprioritized by the consent-as-enthusiasm paradigm, which divides sex into the categories [of] awesome and rape and leaves unaccounted and unaddressed all the immiserating sex too many people, typically women, endure." [1]

Good sex matters because pleasure matters, and that makes bad sex matter. Most human beings are physiologically wired to seek sex, just like we're wired to seek food, and the pleasure we get from it feeds our brain's complicated rewards network. Yet as this book aims to show, the sex-to-pleasure pipeline is out of whack, for an untold number of sexually active young people. As humans, we have made such an enormous, weird deal out of sex—as an institution, as a threat, as a sacrament—that pleasure has taken a back seat. (As author Katherine Angel puts it: "How can sex matter less, so it can yield more?") On one end of the spectrum, you have people who believe sex is so special they save it for their wedding night, which can cause problems, because good sex usually takes practice. On the other end of the spectrum, you have people like me who believe sex is so unremarkable that they dissociate during doggy-style. (In the middle, you have a handful of people with fulfilling, pleasurable sex lives. Happy for them . . .)

What *is* consistent across the sex-having spectrum, what we must immediately understand, is that sex means different things to different people, and there is no correct way to relate to it, as long as you're not bothering other people.

So, is sex, whatever it is, special?

We know that it is, and I can think of one big reason why: pleasure. I'll repeat: good sex matters because pleasure matters, and that makes bad sex matter. Pleasure, a physiological state of being that impacts almost every aspect of our wellness, is a public health issue, and sexual pleasure is a fundamental aspect of sexual health, rights, and well-being. Growing evidence shows that incorporating pleasure into sexual health promotion is more likely to thwart risky behavior, and STI- and HIV-prevention messages have better public health outcomes when they include portrayals of positive sexual experiences. For example, one of the biggest deterrents for condom use is the perception that wearing one will make sex feel worse. Public health campaigns are more effective when they include strategies to increase sexual pleasure while using condoms and other forms of birth control. The Pleasure Project, an advocacy organization founded in 2014 that aims to "eroticize safer sex," trains sex educators to take more sex-positive, pleasure-based approaches.

The ubiquity of social forces that limit, stigmatize, and otherwise criminalize pleasure make sex even more special, more worthy of our attention. Our experience of sex, whether pleasure is present or not, represents a fundamental aspect of our identity.

A recent scandal illuminates just how fraught sex is. Parents of students at the Dalton School in New York City were outraged to discover their first-graders had learned about self-pleasure. During a lesson, sex educator Justine Ang Fonte played an informational cartoon where a boy asks, "Hey, how come sometimes my penis gets big . . . and points in the air?" The video explains what an erection is, and the boy says, "Sometimes I touch my penis because it feels good." A girl adds, "Sometimes, when I'm in my bath or when Mom puts me to bed, I like to touch my vulva, too."

Once the outrage spread from these exorbitantly wealthy parents to right-leaning news media, the backlash was swift and unhinged. Candace Owens tweeted, "A teacher named Justine Fonte taught first-graders via a cartoon about how it feels good when they touch their clitoris and penis. In my opinion, she should have to register as a sex offender. This is worse than woke—it's pedophilic." Several months later, the headmaster announced that Fonte would not be returning to the school. In response, *The Daily Mail* published a story with a headline that read, "Sex-ed teacher at $55,000-per-year NYC private school RESIGNS after angering parents by teaching first-graders about masturbation and telling kids they can't be hugged 'without consent.'"

Months after the scandal, Fonte told me that she was still inundated with hateful emails and DMs, many of them threatening murder. Those messages took up half her inbox. The other half were notes of extreme gratitude; people saying they desperately wished they'd had her as a sex educator when they were children. It struck Fonte that only sex could illicit such polarized, intensely emotional reactions. She posited that the people who want her dead must have been profoundly hurt by sex to be so viscerally triggered by her mission to ensure that young people learn to feel safe and happy in their bodies.

Here is something we all know to be true: children find out about sex. They find out about sex from misinformed peers, and, increasingly, from porn that they are in no way equipped to process. If they receive any sex education at all, they are taught to fear sex, which is presented as a harbinger of disease, pregnancy, and God's wrath. At no point are youth taught that sex should feel good. Fonte, and an increasing number of progressive educators like her, recognize that the absence of pleasure in sexual education is a public health crisis. Not only has pleasure-absent sex ed been shown to leave children more vulnerable to sexual assault, but it sends a clear message that pleasure is not an operative part of the sexual experience. People socialized as women learn young that sex is tolerated for others' benefits, like horny boys, and everyone learns that sex could kill us. When we marginalize pleasure from sex education, we cement lifelong body shame and difficulty asserting sexual autonomy. How can we say yes to what we love and no to what we don't if we haven't learned how? Even first-graders grow up to be sexually active adults, who—if they've learned to feel shame or ambivalence about the pleasure in their own bodies—have horrible sex, again and again. I was that first-grader, and I became that sexually active adult.

Young people deserve to be taught that the pleasure they feel in their bodies is normal—and that it belongs to them and no one else. Why should we insist upon letting little kids think they're perverted freaks for masturbating? When we try to "protect" kids from the realities of sex, we fail them. We won't be able to fix the Bad Sex Problem unless we start young, with squishy brains that absorb everything they see, hear, and intuit about their sexuality.

A growing number of scholars, educators, and activists are working to build a society where access to pleasure, including sexual, is democratized. A recent definition of sexual pleasure, from the Global Advisory Board (GAB) for Sexual Health and Wellbeing, illuminates not only the significance of pleasure in public health, but also just how far we've come: the fact that

GAB and other groups like it exist, to advocate for inclusive, pleasure-centric approaches to sexuality, is remarkable.

> Sexual pleasure is the physical and/or psychological satisfaction and enjoyment derived from solitary or shared erotic experiences, including thoughts, dreams and autoeroticism. Self-determination, consent, safety, privacy, confidence and the ability to communicate and negotiate sexual relations are key enabling factors for pleasure to contribute to sexual health and wellbeing. Sexual pleasure should be exercised within the context of sexual rights, particularly the rights to equality and non-discrimination, autonomy and bodily integrity, the right to the highest attainable standard of health and freedom of expression. The experiences of human sexual pleasure are diverse and sexual rights ensure that pleasure is a positive experience for all concerned and not obtained by violating other people's human rights and wellbeing.[2]

Academic interest in the intersection of pleasure and public health is growing, too, and hopefully it continues to. In 2019, The World Association for Sexual Health Congress issued a Declaration on Sexual Pleasure that explicitly calls for "an intersectional, interdisciplinary and multi-sectorial approach to research, programs, service delivery, and advocacy that fully takes into account the links between sexual health and sexual rights and pleasure." UNESCO now offers guidance on pleasure-informed sexual education. And yet(!), the United States continues to ignore this salient aspect of sexual well-being.

In "The Public Health of Pleasure: Going Beyond Disease Prevention," authors Stewart Landers and Farzana Kapadia remark that the field of sexual health and relationships is increasingly recognizing "that healthy relationships and sexuality are about not merely the absence of sexually transmitted diseases and intimate partner violence but also the presence of pleasurable and satisfying occurrences." They underscore that public health has always been inextricably linked to pleasure. Even the formation of the Environmental Protection Agency, founded to prevent diseases like cholera, typhoid, and emphysema, had a pleasure connection: "There was undeniably pleasure to be had in breathing clean air, drinking purified water, and seeing skies unblackened by smog."

In law, advocacy, health care, and Maria-sexual-decision-making, pleasure should be front and center. Yet it remains marginalized—in both academic circles and the public imagination at large. The Dalton parents are not alone in finding pleasure scandalous and obscene; Fonte's inbox is proof.

I spoke with Dr. Jessie V. Ford, a sociologist and postdoctoral research scientist at Columbia University whose research deals with pleasure and public health. When she was getting her PhD, she recalls being frequently discouraged from studying pleasure. "Don't do pleasure until you get tenure," she remembers a professor saying. "People just won't take you seriously." In the past few years, Ford has published several articles examining the sociological significance of pleasure, including a 2019 paper in the *International Journal of Sexual Health* called "Why Pleasure Matters: Its Global Relevance for Sexual Health, Sexual Rights, and Wellbeing."

"People think pleasure just means we're going to promote everyone having an orgasm, that we're going to teach kids to have orgasms, and it gets really simplified," she said. "They've missed the point that the main reason a lot of people have sex is to connect, to feel pleasure, to feel fulfilled, to feel a deeper, even transcendent emotional meaning. And pleasure, if you interview people about it, encompasses all those things and more."

≈ ≈

Even though our bodies are wired to feel it, pleasure is learned—and unlearned and relearned. At my last session of sex coaching, we finally tackled my genitals. "Your pussy, your vulva, your yoni, whatever you prefer to call it," Weissfeld said, sitting in the back of her van-office. I hated these words. "Pussy" makes me cringe, and "yoni" sounds like a Pokémon or wellness start-up. I was determined to get comfortable with "vulva"—to say "vulva" when I wanted to say "vagina," which would be anatomically imprecise.

We began with a grounding exercise. I closed my eyes and connected to my breath "as an inner lover." Weissfeld asked me to conjure a person or animal that made me feel safe. I imagined my best friend sitting next to me on my couch. We were laughing, eating potato chips, and making disparaging remarks about mutual friends. I felt a warm, melting sensation in my chest.

"The next time you notice tightness or someplace that doesn't feel good in your body, you have this tool," she said. "You have this friend that you can call to your side and allow yourself to lean into this safety. It's an important skill to have as we start to step into something like orgasm. The thing that's so scary about sexuality and orgasm, whether it's by yourself or with somebody else, is this idea of not having control."

She suggested I conjure my friend before masturbating. "It's a way to remember, 'Hey, I can step into the fear. I can take a little step onto the precipice,' but then know that I'm not just going to fall into the pit of despair. I can pull myself back: I get to call my friend to my side, right? Or my dog. Or I can put myself in a place where there are unicorns."

Too many of us never learn to self-soothe, which is unfortunate, because only when we can soothe our overstimulated, undernourished nervous systems does pleasure become possible. There is no specific technique that can turn bad sex into pleasurable sex. There is no new angle or position that can rehabilitate your relationship with pleasure. But there are so many little practices, little shifts in perspectives that can open our bodies up to pleasure—to "orgasmic yeses," as adrienne maree brown calls them. Conjuring my friend before masturbating did, in fact, help me relax enough to feel pleasure in my body. Telling a sexual partner, "Hey, could you lighten the pressure and pick up the pace," did, in fact, help me enjoy myself enough to *approach* the *preliminary* stages of *pre*-orgasm *buildup*. I'm not claiming any one trick will unlock explosive orgasm and save your marriage, or even that either of those two goals are worth pursuing. Rather, I hope this ragtag assortment of tools can help you figure out the type of sex you want to have, the type of sex you don't want to have, and how to pursue the former.

It's a practice—sex, pleasure, all of it. We can resign our-selves to bad sex because the practice feels too tedious; resigning ourselves to anything is our birthright. But our enjoyment of sex matters. Good sex matters. Bad sex matters. Your pleasure matters. And our lives begin to change when we honor what our bodies want, because pleasure is not only a change agent, it's a fundamental human right.

ACKNOWLEDGMENTS

Writing this book during the pandemic took everything out of me, and I couldn't have finished it without the support of such a smart, generous team, starting with my agent, Sharon Pelletier, who tracked me down in 2017 after I wrote a truly deranged piece about eating at the Times Square Olive Garden ten days in a row. Thank you for believing in me and always responding to my Jenna Maroney–esque emails with kind words and crucial perspective. To Sarah Grill, thank you for being the best first-book editor a deeply neurotic person could ask for. Your patience, humor, and eye have been a lifeline to me during this process, and I am so grateful to have found a home at St. Martin's.

The gratitude I feel for the people in my life who have supported me through the writing, editing, fretting, and everything is almost overwhelming. To Holly Gover, Julian Domo, and Burt Reynolds (who came up with the title): your daily support and care have sustained me through this journey, and you are the reasons I could finish this. To Sarah Crowder, Claire Carusillo, Gaby Gutierrez, LGRT, Elsa and Megan, the Delco girlies, and so many more friends who've stuck by me when things got incredibly hard—I love you all and don't know what I would do without you. To every other friend, coworker, and person in my Instagram Story Close Friends who has supported me these past few years, I appreciate you so much for bearing witness to my meltdowns and offering encouragement when I needed it. Thank you to Regan Stephens for driving me to the hospital. Thank you to my family for instilling in me at a young age that being an author was possible and for supporting me every step of the way. Graceanne, thank you for loving Bucatina like family and taking such good care of her when I'm gone.

I am so grateful to every person who spoke to me about their sex life—for this project, and over the years. None of the work I've done would be possible without the unflinching honesty of strangers, acquaintances, and readers. I am also indebted to the researchers, activists, sex workers, and authors, many of whom blessed me with their time and expertise for this book, who have refined and championed so many of the ideas I put forth here. Special thanks to Simone Justice, Aoife Murray, Amy Weissfeld, Dr. Nan Wise, Lucy Sweetkill, Justine Ang Fonte, Carol Queen, adrienne maree brown, Step Tranovich, Julian Gavino, Gabrielle Alexa Noel, Char Adams, and many, many others for being so generous with your time and expertise. Also, shout out to everyone who has had sex with me, including (especially?) the people who have wronged me in some way. I couldn't have done this without you.

Enormous thanks to Bettina Makalintal, Rupa Bhattacharya, Rosa Heyman, Jane Brendlinger, Kat Kinsman, Annabel Kim, Regan, and Holly for early reads; your insight, generosity, and "lol" comments were essential to me and my process as I wrote this in near-total isolation.

To everyone who gave me a blurb: I would die for you. God, thank you.

NOTES

INTRODUCTION

1. "People Think Everyone Is Having a Lot of Sex, But a Survey Shows That's Not the Case," August 9, 2018. https://www.buzzfeednews.com/article/laurenstrapagiel/how-much-sex-is-normal-women-men

2. D. Easton & C. A. Liszt, *The Ethical Slut: A Guide to Infinite Sexual Possibilities* (San Francisco, CA: Greenery Press, 1997).

1: THE SEX RECESSION AND ITS HIDDEN PROMISE

1. Michael Dimock, "Defining Generations," Pew Research Center (2019). https://www.pewresearch.org/fact-tank/2019/01/17/where-millennials-end-and-generation-z-begins/

2. "Trends in Ages at Key Reproductive Transitions in the United States, 1951–2010," *Women's Health Issues* 2014, May–Jun; 24(3): e271–e279. https://www.ncbi.nlm.nih.gov/pmc/articles/PMC4011992/

3. Richard Fry, "The share of Americans living without a partner has increased, especially among young adults," Pew Research Center (2017). https://www.pewresearch.org/fact-tank/2017/10/11/the-share-of-americans-living-without-a-partner-has-increased-especially-among-young-adults/

4. "Queer People See More Harassment in Dating Apps Than Straights," Pew Research Center, (2020). https://www.advocate.com/love-and-sex/2020/5/19/queer-people-see-more-harassment-dating-apps-straights

5. "Tinder Still Banning Transgender People Despite Pledge of Inclusivity," *The Independent* (2019) https://www.independent.co.uk /news/world/americas/tinder-ban-trans-account-block-report-lawsuit -pride-gender-identity-a9007721.html

6. "Singles' Sexual Satisfaction Is Associated with More Satisfaction With Singlehood and Less Interest in Marriage," *Personality and Social Psychology Bulletin,* August 11, 2020.

2: THE BAD SEX PROBLEM

1. *Didactic Poetry of Greece, Rome and Beyond: Knowledge, Power, Tradition,* 239. Translation by Willis Barnstone. Edited by Lilah Grace Canevaro, and Donncha O'Rourke: Classic Press of Wales, 2019.

2. "Babylonian terracotta plaque with erotic scene," Barakat Gallery. http://store.barakatgallery.com/product/babylonian-terracotta-plaque -erotic-scene/

3. James Lambert, "Ancient Mesopotamian Erotic Art," 2019. https://medium.com/@jameslambert537/ancient-mesopotamian-erotic -art-989d2df92fe

4. https://www.buzzfeednews.com/article/madeleineholden/gen-z -sex-positivity

5. M. É. Czeisler, R. I. Lane & E. Petrosky, et al., "Mental Health, Substance Use, and Suicidal Ideation During the COVID-19 Pandemic—United States, June 24–30, 2020." *MMWR Morb Mortal Wkly Rep* 2020; 69:1049–1057. DOI: http://dx.doi.org/10.15585/mmwr .mm6932a1external icon

6. K. Rømer Thomsen, P. C. Whybrow & M. L Kringelbach (2015). "Reconceptualizing anhedonia: novel perspectives on balancing the pleasure networks in the human brain," *Frontiers in Behavioral Neuroscience* 9: 49. doi:10.3389/fnbeh.2015.00049. PMC 4356228. PMID 25814941

7. "The Neural Correlates of Anhedonia in Major Depressive Disorder," *Biological Psychiatry* 58, no. 11 (2005): 843–53.

8. "Mental health issues increased significantly in young adults over last decade," March 19, 2019, American Psychological Association. https://www.sciencedaily.com/releases/2019/03/190315110908.htm

9. "Mental Health, Substance Use, and Suicidal Ideation During the COVID-19 Pandemic—United States, June 24–30, 2020," Morbidity and Mortality Weekly Report, Center for Disease Control and Prevention, August 14, 2020. https://www.cdc.gov/mmwr/volumes/69/wr/mm6932a1.htm?s_cid=mm6932a1_w#contribAff

10. "Labia Problems," https://www.healthdirect.gov.au/labia-problems.

11. https://www.grid.news/story/politics/2022/08/27/book-banning-in-us-schools-has-reached-an-all-time-high-what-this-means-and-how-we-got-here/

12. https://www.plannedparenthood.org/planned-parenthood-st-louis-region-southwest-missouri/blog/that-8-letter-word-including-pleasure-in-sex-education

13. "Sex and HIV Education," November 1, 2020. Guttmacher Institute. https://www.guttmacher.org/state-policy/explore/sex-and-hiv-education

14. "Implicit Puritanism in American moral cognition," *Journal of Experimental Social Psychology* 47(2) March 2011, 312–320. https://www.sciencedirect.com/science/article/abs/pii/S0022103110002301

15. "How Evangelical Purity Culture Can Lead to a Lifetime of Sexual Shame," Vice.com, October 16, 2018. https://www.vice.com/en/article/pa98x8/purity-culture-linday-kay-klein-pure-review

16. J. K. Tran, G. Dunckel & E. J. Teng. "Sexual dysfunction in veterans with post-traumatic stress disorder." *J Sex Med* 2015 Apr; 12(4): 847–55. doi: 10.1111/jsm.12823. Epub 2015 Feb 9. PMID: 25665140.

17. "The Role of Sexual Communication in Couples' Sexual Outcomes: A Dyadic Path Analysis," *Journal of Marital and Family Therapy* 44(4) October 2018: 606–23.

18. E. A. Babin (2013). "An examination of predictors of nonverbal and verbal communication of pleasure during sex and sexual satisfaction." *Journal of Social and Personal Relationships* 30(3), 270–92.

3: CYBERSEX LIVES

1. J. Firth, J. Torous & B. Stubbs, et al. "The 'online brain': how the internet may be changing our cognition, *World Psychiatry* 2019; 18(2): 119–29. doi:10.1002/wps.20617

2. https://www.theguardian.com/technology/2018/may/08/social-media-copies-gambling-methods-to-create-psychological-cravings

3. L. Y. Lin, J. E. Sidani & A. Shensa. "Association between social media use and depression among U.S. young adults," *Depression Anxiety* 2016; 33: 323–31.

4. Nan Wise, *Why Good Sex Matters.* Harvest (January 28, 2020).

5. https://www.wsj.com/articles/facebook-knows-instagram-is-toxic-for-teen-girls-company-documents-show-11631620739

6. https://guilfordjournals.com/doi/10.1521/jscp.2018.37.10.751

7. Y. L. Reid Chassiakos, J. Radesky, D. Christakis, M. A. Moreno & C. Cross. Council on Communications and Media. "Children and Adolescents and Digital Media." *Pediatrics* 2016 Nov; 138(5): e20162593. doi: 10.1542/peds.2016–2593. PMID: 27940795.

8. "Bye-bye booty: Heroin chic is back," *New York Post,* November 2, 2022. nypost. com/2022/11/02/heroin-chic-is-back-and-curvy-bodies-big-butts-are-out/

9. K. E. Baker (2016). "Online pornography: Should schools be teaching young people about the risks? An exploration of the views of young people and teaching professionals." *Sex Education* 16(2), 213–28. doi:10.1080/14681811.2015.1090968

10. https://www.npr.org/2019/05/25/723192364/what-we-dont-talk-about-when-we-talk-about-porn

11. https://www.apa.org/news/press/releases/2017/08/pornography-exposure

12. https://journals.sagepub.com/doi/10.1177/2056305117738992

4: THE POWER OF SEX CLEANSES, DRY SPELLS, AND AVOIDING SEX ALTOGETHER

1. Josiah Hesse, "Growing Up Evangelical Ruined Sex for Me," *Vice,* October 8, 2018. https://www.vice.com/en/article/neg958/growing-up-evangelical-ruined-sex-for-me

2. Sandra Vilarinhoa, *Current Opinion in Psychiatry* 30(6) November 2017, 402–08(7), DOI: https://doi.org/10.1097/YCO.0000000000000363

3. Lori A. Brotto and Rosemary Basson. "Group mindfulness-based

therapy significantly improves sexual desire in women," *Behaviour Research and Therapy,* vol. 57, 2014, 43–54, ISSN 0005–7967, https://doi.org/10.1016/j.brat.2014.04.001 http://www.sciencedirect.com/science/article/pii/S0005796714000497

4. J. A. Bossio, R. Basson, M. Driscoll, S. Correia & L. A. Brotto. "Mindfulness-Based Group Therapy for Men with Situational Erectile Dysfunction: A Mixed-Methods Feasibility Analysis and Pilot Study." *J Sex Med* 2018 Oct; 15(10): 1478–90. doi: 10.1016/j.jsxm.2018.08.013. PMID: 30297094.

5. Steve Stewart-Williams, Caroline A. Butler & Andrew G. Thomas (2017) "Sexual History and Present Attractiveness: People Want a Mate with a Bit of a Past, But Not Too Much," *The Journal of Sex Research* 54(9) 1097–105, DOI: 10.1080/00224499.2016.1232690

6. B. J. Willoughby & J. Vitas. "Sexual desire discrepancy: the effect of individual differences in desired and actual sexual frequency on dating couples," *Arch Sex Behav* 2012 Apr; 41(2): 477–86. doi: 10.1007/s10508-011-9766-9. Epub 2011 May 14. PMID: 21573707.

7. Katherine Rowland (2020). *The Pleasure Gap: American Women and the Unfinished Sexual Revolution,* Seal Press, February 4, 2020, p. 43.

5: THE TRANSFORMATIVE
POWER OF MASTURBATION

1. G. Castellini, E. Fanni, G. Corona, E. Maseroli, V. Ricca, & M. Maggi (2016). "Psychological, Relational, and Biological Correlates of Ego-Dystonic Masturbation in a Clinical Setting," *Sexual Medicine* 4(3), e156–e165. https://doi.org/10.1016/j.esxm.2016.03.024

2. Christine Kaestle & Katherine Allen (2011). "The Role of Masturbation in Healthy Sexual Development: Perceptions of Young Adults," *Archives of Sexual Behavior* 40, 983–94. 10.1007/s10508-010-9722-0.

3. B. D. Zamboni & I. Crawford. "Using masturbation in sex therapy," *Journal of Psychology & Human Sexuality* 2003; 14(2–3): 123–41. doi: 10.1300/J056v14n02_08.

4. A. O. Sasmita, J. Kuruvilla & A. P. Ling (November 2018). "Harnessing neuroplasticity: modern approaches and clinical future," *The*

International Journal of Neuroscience, 128(11): 1061–77. doi:10.1080/002 07454.2018.1466781. PMID 29667473. S2CID 4957270.

6: I GOT A SEX COACH

1. Thomas Maier, *Masters of Sex: The Life and Times of William Masters and Virginia Johnson, the Couple Who Taught America How to Love,* Basic Books, July 30, 2013, p. 212.

2. Shere Hite, *The Hite Report: A Nationwide Study of Female Sexuality* (Seven Stories Press, 2004).

3. M. Loe, *The Rise of Viagra: How the Little Blue Pill Changed Sex in America* (NYU Press, 2004).

4. Katherine Rowland, *The Pleasure Gap: American Women and the Unfinished Sexual Revolution* (Seal Press, 2020).

5. M. Berner & C. Günzler (2012). "Efficacy of psychosocial interventions in men and women with sexual dysfunctions—a systematic review of controlled clinical trials." *The Journal of Sexual Medicine,* 9, 3089–107. doi:10.1111/j.1743-6109.2012.02970.

6. L. A. Brotto, Y. Erskine, M. Carey, T. Ehlen, S. Finlayson, M. Heywood, J. Kwon, J. McAlpine, G. Stuart, S. Thomson, & D. Miller. "A brief mindfulness-based cognitive behavioral intervention improves sexual functioning versus wait-list control in women treated for gynecologic cancer," *Gynecol Oncol* 2012 May; 125(2): 320–5. doi: 10.1016/j.ygyno.2012.01.035. Epub 2012 Jan 28. PMID: 22293042; PMCID: PMC3438201.

7. M. Meyers, J. Margraf & J. Velten. "Psychological Treatment of Low Sexual Desire in Women: Protocol for a Randomized, Waitlist-Controlled Trial of Internet-Based Cognitive Behavioral and Mindfulness-Based Treatments," *JMIR Res Protoc* 2020 Sep 29; 9(9): e20326. doi: 10.2196/20326. PMID: 32990248; PMCID: PMC7556380.

8. C. Caizzi. "Embodied Trauma: Using the Subsymbolic Mode to Access and Change Script Protocol in Traumatized Adults," *Transactional Analysis Journal,* 2012; 42(3): 165–75. doi:10.1177 /036215371204200302.

9. Katherine Rowland, *The Pleasure Gap.*

10. "The Future of Well-Being in a Tech-Saturated World." Pew Research Center, April 2018. https://assets.pewresearch.org/wp-content /uploads/sites/14/2018/04/14154552/PI_2018.04.17_Future-of-Well -Being_FINAL.pdf

11. Russell M. Viner, et al. "Roles of cyberbullying, sleep, and physical activity in mediating the effects of social media use on mental health and wellbeing among young people in England: a secondary analysis of longitudinal data." *The Lancet Child & Adolescent Health,* 3(10) 685–96.

8: TOY STORY

1. https://www.nytimes.com/2020/06/07/style/sex-toys-online -coronavirus.html

2. M. Dewitte & Y. Reisman. "Clinical use and implications of sexual devices and sexually explicit media," *Nat Rev Urol* 18, 359–77 (2021). https://doi.org/10.1038/s41585-021-00456-2

3. C. A. Graham (2014). "Orgasm disorders in women" in Y. M. Binik & K. S. K. Hall (Eds.), *Principles and Practice of Sex Therapy* (5th ed.,) (New York, NY: The Guilford Press, 89–111).

4. M. J. Stein, H. Lin & R. Wang. "New advances in erectile technology," *Ther Adv Urol* 2014 Feb; 6(1) 15–24.

5. https://www.thecut.com/2017/11/the-30-000-year-history-of -the-sex-toy.html

6. Ibid.

7. https://www.grandviewresearch.com/industry-analysis/sex-toys -market

8. https://thatshandi.co/pages/about-us

9: COMMUNICATION 101

1. Allen B. Mallory, Amelia M. Stanton & Ariel B. Handy (2019). "Couples' Sexual Communication and Dimensions of Sexual Function:

A Meta-Analysis," *The Journal of Sex Research* 56(7) 882–98, DOI: 10.1080/00224499.2019.1568375

2. U. S. Rehman, D. Balan, S. Sutherland & J. McNeil. "Understanding barriers to sexual communication," *Journal of Social and Personal Relationships,* 2019; 36(9): 2605–23. doi:10.1177/0265407518794900

3. bell hooks, *All About Love,* William Morrow Paperbacks, January 30, 2018, p. 3.

4. S. F. Dingfelder (2011, April). "Understanding orgasm," *Monitor on Psychology* 42(4). http://www.apa.org/monitor/2011/04/orgasm

5. E. A. Harris, M. J. Hornsey, H. F. Larsen, et al. "Beliefs About Gender Predict Faking Orgasm in Heterosexual Women," *Arch Sex Behav* 48, 2419–33 (2019). https://doi.org/10.1007/s10508-019-01510-2

6. L. J. Séguin & R. R. Milhausen (2016). "Not all fakes are created equal: examining the relationships between men's motives for pretending orgasm and levels of sexual desire, and relationship and sexual satisfaction," *Sexual and Relationship Therapy* 31(2) 159–75.

7. C. L. Muehlenhard & S. K. Shippee (2010). "Men's and Women's Reports of Pretending Orgasm," *Journal of Sex Research* 46, 1–16.

8. "Co-Dependency," Mental Health America. https://www.mhanational.org/co-dependency

9. Martin, *The Art of Receiving and Giving,* p. 27.

10. http://www.haileymagee.com/blog/2021/1/8/the-recovering-people-pleasers-guide-to-empowered-sexual-intimacy

11. Laurie Mintz, *Becoming Cliterate,* HarperOne, May 9, 2017, p. 163.

CONCLUSION

1. Joseph Fischel, *Screw Consent: A Better Politics of Sexual Justice,* University of California Press, January 2019, p. 4.

2. Global Advisory Board for Sexual Health and Wellbeing: c2006–2018. Working definition of sexual pleasure; 2016 [cited 2018 Mar 24]. Available from: http://www.gab-shw.org/our-work/working-definition-of-sexual-pleasure/

INDEX

·